ROUTLEDGE LIBRARY EDITIONS:
MARRIAGE

Volume 7

SEX BEFORE MARRIAGE

SEX BEFORE MARRIAGE

ELEANOR HAMILTON

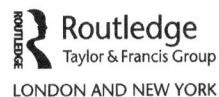
LONDON AND NEW YORK

First published in Great Britain in 1971 by
George Allen & Unwin Ltd

This edition first published in 2023
by Routledge
4 Park Square, Milton Park, Abingdon, Oxon OX14 4RN

and by Routledge
605 Third Avenue, New York, NY 10158

Routledge is an imprint of the Taylor & Francis Group, an informa business

© 1969 Eleanor Hamilton

All rights reserved. No part of this book may be reprinted or reproduced or utilised in any form or by any electronic, mechanical, or other means, now known or hereafter invented, including photocopying and recording, or in any information storage or retrieval system, without permission in writing from the publishers.

Trademark notice: Product or corporate names may be trademarks or registered trademarks, and are used only for identification and explanation without intent to infringe.

British Library Cataloguing in Publication Data
A catalogue record for this book is available from the British Library

ISBN: 978-1-032-46071-0 (Set)
ISBN: 978-1-032-47898-2 (Volume 7) (hbk)
ISBN: 978-1-032-47918-7 (Volume 7) (pbk)
ISBN: 978-1-003-38652-0 (Volume 7) (ebk)

DOI: 10.4324/9781003386520

Publisher's Note
The publisher has gone to great lengths to ensure the quality of this reprint but points out that some imperfections in the original copies may be apparent.

Disclaimer
The publisher has made every effort to trace copyright holders and would welcome correspondence from those they have been unable to trace.

Language Disclaimer
This book is a re-issue originally published in 1969.
The language used and views portrayed are a reflection of its era and no offence is meant by the Publishers to any reader by this re-publication.

New Preface to the Reissue of 2023
Sex Before Marriage

Sex Before Marriage—first published in March 1969, two years after the famous "summer of love," was not, for most young people, an introduction to the notion of premarital sex. Premarital sex was a fact of American life, albeit one still buried under layers of hypocrisy and silence. What young people *did* gain by the book's publication was some practical advice from an adult sympathetic to their situation. One reviewer in 1970 noted that although the author of *Sex Before Marriage* was "an experienced psychologist," the book still managed to be "remarkably free of that profession's jargon or theoretical biases. It is doubtful that youngsters would classify [the] book as 'far out,' but they are certain to label Dr. Hamilton's work as being 'with it.'"

This reprinted edition, arriving in 2023, provides an opportunity to appraise how much has changed since 1969, and how much hasn't.

Hamilton's main regret in the years following this book's publication was its treatment of homosexuality—tellingly included here in a chapter titled "Sexual Deviancy." She was a woman struggling to keep her professional credibility in the pathbreaking work of introducing sex positivity to McCarthy era America. It is likely that, in this context, she did not wish to wander even further beyond the pale by questioning the culture's homophobia. It leads her into inconsistencies. For the teen considering premarital sex, Hamilton offers a list of questions to help the reader find their own moral conscience rather than bow to an outdated cultural norm ("Does my sexual activity harm anyone?") Meanwhile the gay reader "would do well to consult a therapist, for while homosexuality is not a disease it is a condition that is likely to isolate you from the vast majority of other people." Her treatment eschews medically pathologizing same sex attraction, but it clearly lacks the courage of conscience apparent elsewhere in the book.

By 1978 both Dr. Hamilton and the times had evolved enough that, in *Sex, with Love: A Guide For Young People,* she writes in the chapter on "Same Sex Relationships" "I like to define sex as energy—a special kind of energy that tends to draw us one to another for companionship, love, physical closeness, body pleasure, and sometimes procreation...And this is true whether the love we bear is for man, woman, child, nature, or what some people call god." She offers some guarded encouragement for those considering pursuing a same-sex relationship openly: "In this, as in other things, it takes a brave and committed person to do something that society frowns on." In a 1996 interview she opened up still further, sharing her own experience of sexual relationships with other women: "If I had to identify myself I would call myself bisexual... But then, I think everybody is bisexual. I don't like those categories. I believe we love who we love." In her 2000 preface to *Still Doing It: Women & Men Over 60 Write About Their Sexuality,* she goes so far as to positively *recommend* same sex relationships to straight women as a practical measure, promising "what an enlivening love life a widow or widower may yet experience in their final years as they open their minds and hearts to the potential fulfillment of same sex love."

After devoting chapters to sexual development, non-coital sex, the "art of first intercourse", and birth control, two chapters: "What can you do if you're pregnant?" and "Going through a pregnancy unwed" address the very real facts of unwanted pregnancy in a country where abortion was illegal.

On January 22, 1973, four years after the book's publication, the US Supreme Court ruling in Roe vs. Wade decriminalized abortion. Readers who wished to terminate pregnancies would no longer have to scour Dr. Hamilton's chapters for information on how to attain a legal abortion in Japan with a note from an American doctor, or how to arrange for an adoption that would allow the biological mother to meet the adoptive parents. Sadly, grotesquely, these chapters directed to the young pregnant person of half a century ago have attained new relevance. Nearly 50 years after Roe enshrined the right to abortion, the U.S. Supreme Court overturned Roe in Dobbs v. Ferguson on June 24, 2022. The reprinting of this book is an opportunity, then, not only to rejoice in "how far we've come" but to observe history's stunning cyclicality within a culture where disavowal of female bodily autonomy dies hard.

The reader familiar with 20th century psychoanalytic history will note the heavy imprint throughout this book of psychoanalyst Wilhelm Reich, and particularly his concept of "muscular armoring." The exercise Dr. Hamilton offers readers in Chapter 4, geared towards achieving a free flow of energy through the body, is condensed Reichean therapy. Dispensed here in a no-nonsense manner alongside instructions on how to choose a pediatrician, pick a hospital, or get a boy's attention, Hamilton puts Reich to practical use. Dr. Hamilton and her husband were patients, students, and ultimately friends of Wilhelm Reich. Reflecting on Reich's troubling final years, Hamilton wrote that part of what destroyed him was the rejection of his ideas by smallminded people. As for herself, introducing radical sexual theories in Cold War America had made her no stranger to persecution. "Certainly", she wrote:

> whenever I have been out on the cutting edge of an idea that has proven right and reasonable and sane, eventually I have met with inexplicable resistance that

sometimes has taken violent form. For example, *when I wrote Sex Before Marriage: Guidance for Young Adults Ages 16–20,* I not only received anonymous threatening telephone calls in which the callers informed me that New Englanders knew how to deal with its witches, but I was also threatened with the burning of my house and warned that I would be tied to a pole and dunked in our pond to determine, as the witch hunter did of yore, my innocence or guilt before God. I have also been visited by religious fanatics who came to "save my soul." I have received dozens of letters imploring me to turn to God, as well as letters asking me to write to libraries requesting that they put my books under lock and key so that children would not be contaminated by them.

Unlike Reich, however, Dr. Hamilton was not interested in becoming a martyr. She coolly noted the ratio of accolades and accusations as it changed over the years to include more of the latter.

Back in 1969, 1 out of every 4 letters I received was damming. By 1982, only 1 in 20 twenty was negative. In fact, the American Library Association paid me the highest compliment in listing my book, *Sex with Love: A Guide for Teenagers,* among the best 40 books of the year for young readers. And after appearing on television shows such as The Today Show and Woman to Woman, as well as being the guest of hosts like Phil Donahue and Merv Griffen and many others, did my ideas receive overwhelmingly more positive responses than negative ones. Does this mean there is a growing body of persons unafraid of the "little men" of whom Reich spoke? And if so, will they develop the strength to oppose those who would deprive us of our right to deep happiness? Or will these "little men" blow up the earth before mankind as a whole can know the full joy of human ecstasy? I wonder!

While there are moments in this book that sounds hopelessly old fashioned, there is much that still feels very fresh: like the idea of releasing anger stored before attempting intimacy, or the concept that sexuality is present in some form in people of all ages, and various stages of life bring various appropriate forms of expression for that energy. She is at perhaps her most timeless when writing about a timeless question: the relationship between sex and love. She advises against loveless sex not on moral grounds but grounds of pleasure: it has diminishing returns, she argues, when not an expression of the creative powers of love.

Sofi Thanhauser
November 2022

SEX BEFORE MARRIAGE

Dr Eleanor Hamilton was born in Portland, Oregon. After obtaining a degree in psychology at the University of Oregon, she became director of a programme for teenage girls at the YWCA. While directing a private school in New York City with her husband she obtained M.A. and Ph.D. degrees from Columbia University.

In addition to her work as a certified psychologist and marriage counsellor, Dr Hamilton lectures at colleges and medical schools and has written many articles for magazines. In 1961 she published her previous book, *Partners in Love*.

Fellow of the American Association of Marriage Counsellors and a member of the American Council of Family Relations, Dr Hamilton is the mother of four children and lives and works in both Massachusetts and New York.

ELEANOR HAMILTON Ph.D.

SEX BEFORE MARRIAGE

Eleanor Hamilton, Ph.D.

LONDON · UNWIN BOOKS

First published in Great Britain in 1971

This book is copyright under the Berne Convention. All rights are reserved. Apart from any fair dealing for the purpose of private study, research, criticism or review, as permitted under the Copyright Act, 1965, no part of this publication may be reproduced, stored in a retrieval system, or transmitted, in any form or by any means, electronic, electrical, chemical, mechanical, optical, photocopying, recording or otherwise, without the prior permission of the copyright owner. Enquiries should be addressed to the publishers.

© 1969 Eleanor Hamilton

UNWIN BOOKS
George Allen & Unwin Ltd
40 Museum Street
London WC1

ISBN 0 04 612022 X Cased
ISBN 0 04 612023 8 Paper

Printed in Great Britain
in 10 point Plantin type
by Clarke, Doble & Brendon Ltd
Plymouth

FOREWORD

IN her work as a psychotherapist Dr Hamilton has gained a remarkable insight into the sexual needs and opportunities of young Americans, with whom she evidently comes into intimate contact. She understands their points of view, the degrees of liberty allowed them in their contemporary social conditions, and the resulting dangers that can occur when this liberty is not wisely used. The frankness and optimism of her own expressed opinions will surely have a wide and healthy influence on all her readers of whatsoever country.

In presenting this book to English readers various changes have been made, such as the replacement of English names and addresses for equivalent American ones when there are in England bodies with similar functions. Similarly, passages describing American hospital conditions and American abortion law, names of books published in America and certain other passages have been altered as necessary, except where the facts and information are interesting in themselves. In the Bibliography both American and British books are listed.

Helena Wright

PUBLISHERS' NOTE

The Publishers would like to thank Mrs Margaret Bramall of the National Council for the Unmarried Mother and Her Child and Dr Helena Wright for their help in preparing the British edition of the chapters relating specifically to pregnancy outside marriage (Chapters 6 and 7), and Mr Eugene Feldman for permission to reproduce his lithograph 'Woman No. 1' on the cover of the British Edition.

PREFACE

THIS book has been written with the hope that it may help young people of college age to use their healthy sexuality for good ends, for self-renewal, for enrichment of body and spirit.

We are born as sexual creatures and our sexuality is a vital force nourishing us throughout life, capable of inspiring creativity and happiness on every level. It is also the force which draws us, one to the other, in comradeship, compassion, friendship, love.

The most important single fact for parents of college-age youth to understand is that sexuality and intercourse are *not* synonymous nor does the one necessarily lead to the other. Too often adults mistakenly believe in the equations:

sexuality = intercourse
premarital intercourse = promiscuity

Both are wrong, and belief in them can lead only to repressive attitudes which, in turn, create sick sexuality.

Intercourse is simply one act among many expressing sexuality. Though intercourse may well be the most involving act in the sexual spectrum, it does not, by any means, embrace all of sexuality. It is only one small, though significant, part of the sexual scene – a part generally reserved for adults who are mature enough to assume the full responsibility implicit in it. Most often this responsibility involves marriage, but always it involves ability to handle the potentiality of birth – and its control.

Sexuality has many expressions not necessarily leading to intercourse. These may range from the tender gestures of affection between mother and child to the equally tender ministrations of old man to old woman as they care for each other toward the end of a meaningful life.

Sexuality can be, and is, a powerful force for good in the world. It can also be perverted to evil purpose, though it is not evil in and of itself.

We have come a long way from Victorian days when many of

the concepts expressed here would have appalled some parents and enraged others. But I am convinced that the vast majority of thoughtful mothers and fathers who have reflected upon the sexual phenomena of man in today's world will realize the necessity for a clearer view of the subject. They will sigh with relief that the still limited knowledge of sex we have obtained is now beginning to be brought out into the open for the enlightenment of young people and for discussion and further research.

Even a sympathetic parent may not agree with all of my conclusions or with my methods of approach to sexual expression. However, I believe that this book will be of service to you as well as to your college-age sons and daughters, as you discuss together the bewildering changes in attitudes that have emerged in the past ten years.

I know, for instance, that it is hard for you to realize that research in the United States shows that one-third of all girls there under thirty today have experienced a premarital pregnancy. This is a preventable tragedy, but it will not be prevented by a conspiracy of silence about noncoital methods of sexual expression and about birth control. Noncoital sexuality has always been with us, but the young do not ordinarily learn of it till after rather than before having had intercourse. Why don't they?

Birth control has been revolutionized by "the pill", and with this technological advance the last social deterrent to premarital intercourse has vanished. Yet the young are often not given instruction in the use of birth control until after rather than before they have had an unwanted pregnancy. Why is this?

The other great deterrent to premarital intercourse, venereal disease, is fast coming under control but remains a serious problem where insufficient care is given to personal hygiene and health, and where relationships are treated irresponsibly.

I also realize how difficult it is for you to feel really relaxed when discussing such natural functions as masturbation or mutual petting to orgasm. The difficulty comes primarily because we have been brainwashed to believe the false equation that sex and intercourse are one and the same, that the one leads inevitably to the other. These equations are not true. In fact, human beings can learn to enjoy the full limits of the sexuality imposed by their chronological age, their physiological age, and their psychological age without intercourse. Furthermore, intercourse is not at many stages of life the most pleasurable or desirable form of sexual expression. At any time, however, there will be *some* form of expression that *is* desirable and appropriate. Life without sexuality would be deadly – but life without intercourse at certain stages of development is not only possible but to be recommended.

Though we do not yet know what is the full range of appropriate sexual activity for various ages, at least we have some clear guideposts that have stood the test of human experience. If our young people have moved into inappropriate or premature forms of sexual expression, it is because they have not been told of appropriate ones, actually more satisfying. Few adults realize that masturbation, for example, can be good, not bad. Even fewer have indicated to youth the varied ways by which satisfaction can be gained in noncoital sexuality. Who tells them of the joy of simple body closeness? The reason is that nearly everyone fears that such acts will lead to only one thing – intercourse, and that this will lead to promiscuity and moral degradation.

The thesis of this book is that expressions of sexuality, if properly understood and permitted, will generally do just the opposite. They will lead to the discovery and practice of ethical forms of sexuality most fulfilling for the age and development of any given individual. If the focus is on intercourse alone, other necessary steps tend to be neglected in the educational process, steps essential to satisfactory sexuality in adult life. As a result, the young person's confidence in his own sexual performance may later suffer, and produce sexual imbalances and deviations.

If any of you could sit day after day as I do, listening to the woes of men and women who have suffered sexual crippling because of this lack of instruction and thus have walked into marriage handicapped, you would say with me that the much touted, so-called "moral law" is actually one of the most immoral principles ever foisted on a gullible public.

Denial of the pleasure principle, which is the basis of happiness in life, leads to frustration, envy, and punitive destructiveness. The end result can only be symptoms of mental and physical illness for your children.

It is up to those of us who have somehow muddled through to sexual fulfilment, despite our upbringing, to clear a better path for the young, to share with them what we know of the ethics of sexuality, remembering that it is not what we know that hurts us, but what we do *not* know.

E.H.

CONTENTS

	page
FOREWORD	v
PUBLISHERS' NOTE	v
PREFACE	vii
1 *How Sexuality Develops*	1
2 *Noncoital Sex*	12
3 *Premarital Intercourse – Pro and Con*	25
4 *The Art of First Intercourse*	34
5 *Birth Control*	41
6 *What Can You Do if You're Pregnant?*	53
7 *If You Decide to Go Through a Pregnancy Unmarried*	71
8 *Sexual Problems*	95
9 *Sexual Deviations*	104
10 *What Professional Help Can You Get?*	111
11 *What of Love?*	120
APPENDIX	
A *Reproductive Biology – A Brief Review*	131
B *Bibliography*	144
C *Some Useful Addresses*	148
INDEX	151

CHAPTER 1

How Sexuality develops

Sex may not be what makes the world go round, but it certainly is what makes the human race keep going. Without it we would not experience one of the greatest pleasures known to man, and without it people would not have children. As you know, you, yourself, owe your very existence to sex. The love your mother and father had for each other started because they were sexually attracted to each other.

Love and sex, however, are not identical. Too many people make the mistake of thinking that they are. Marriages consummated on this assumption tend to go wrong, for while all love does have sexual roots, not all sexual roots sprout forth into love. In other words, all of us are sexual, but not all of us are loving.

Sex is also energy. It is that kind of energy which stirs you and me and everyone to desire closeness to other human beings. It does, in fact, draw all manner of life forms to seek each other, for contact, for pleasure, for comfort, and to reproduce their kind.

Whenever love and sex are connected, people feel deeply contented and are concerned for the well-being of each other. This leads to healthy growth in personality. When love and sex are disconnected, personality tends to suffer in one way or another.

In other words, when your own sexuality is a true expression of your capacity to love, and when it is in accord with your personal system of ethics, you can count on finding happiness. Furthermore, there are ethical and satisfying forms of sexual expression for every age and stage of life.

Actually you have been living with a sexual self ever since you were born, and you will be living with that sexual self until the day you die. Without being aware of it perhaps, you have already had many experiences which were sexual in nature. As you read this chapter, which may seem elementary to those of you who are familiar with the facts of child development, think about your own life. Parts of it you will not be able to recall, but some of the things I say here may stir your memory and help you to understand your present attitudes about sex.

Actually the sexual development of each of us begins the moment we are conceived. We remember nothing about this, of course, because at the moment we were nothing more than an infinitesimal sperm from our father's penis meeting with the tiniest egg descending the Fallopian tube to the womb of our mother. But the way our mother and father felt about creating us, and their love for each other at the time, had a profound effect upon our development.

Doctors now know that the mother who wants a child carries that child inside her with a pleasurable awareness of his being that helps her to relax and enjoy her pregnancy. Her relaxation also allows the developing baby a maximum amount of freedom to move within her body. As he moves he is, of course, exercising and as you must have guessed, the baby who exercises most also develops most.

There is evidence that some form of nonverbal communication goes on between mother and baby while the baby is still inside the mother. For example, she can press upon her abdomen and is likely to get in response a kick of a tiny foot or a thrust of a wee fist.

If she was trained for childbirth, she learned how to anticipate the involuntary movements of her muscles as her baby was thrust out into the world. Furthermore, she co-operated in this birth with love. By her knowledge and co-operation she helped her baby get through the most traumatic experience he will ever know. If the mother was not anaesthetized at the moment of birth, she welcomed her baby with her whole conscious being. As soon as he drew breath and his cord was tied and cut, she snuggled him close to her warm body. This closeness of body is perhaps the first direct sexual experience that anyone has. An infant's "reach out" to life is probably by way of his mouth, and one of the early sexual things he does is to put his thumb in his mouth and suck. Sucking is comforting and pleasurable to him.

You may think it strange that I call sucking a sexual act – but if you keep in mind that we are defining as sexual all those processes which bring us body pleasure or body comfort and draw us one to the other, you will understand why I have called sucking "sexual". Actually, much of infantile sucking serves no other purpose than to give the baby pleasure and comfort.

In a baby's contact with his mother's breast, or in being held close while she gives him a bottle, he takes in more than milk when he suckles. He absorbs, as well, the intangible thing we call a sense of being loved, which she, his mother, quite tangibly expresses to him through this warm body contact. The chances are that he feels comfortable all over when he finds her welcoming breast and that he experiences the world as a responsive and hospitable place.

His breathing resembles that of a contented puppy with the emphasis on exhalation, not inhalation. Already what we call the *orgasm reflex* is in operation. In other words, each time he breathes out, he feels a pleasurable streaming sensation coursing through his body from his centre to his extremities. His trunk forms a slight curve each time he exhales.

Then, with each inhalation his trunk straightens, ever so little, and with each exhalation it collapses again into a gentle curve. This hardly perceptible but unbroken flow of pleasurable movement forms the base of the orgasm reflex. Later on in life if a person wants full enjoyment of sex, it is important that this reflex be as healthy as possible.

You may ask, "What is an orgasm, anyway?"

This is a word that you will hear again and again. Later on in this book I will talk more about the orgasm, but for now let me say simply that when any of the erotic areas of the body, most specifically the sexual organs, are stimulated pleasurably so that they become engorged, and the individual feels that he cannot further contain the tension, his whole organism seems to explode in a kind of convulsion which rocks his body from head to toes, and then subsides, leaving him relaxed – and usually at peace with himself and the world.

In the past the word orgasm was used almost exclusively to signify the culmination of sexual intercourse. But in recent years its use has been extended to include manifestations of the orgasm reflex at all levels of development.

If you could see an orgasm operating in a baby, it would appear as a wavelike movement. Then you would notice a momentary quivering, and shortly after, the baby would lie quietly relaxed, usually dropping off to sleep.

Most mothers do not recognize an orgasm in an infant. Therefore, they react with astonishment when scientists tell them that even quite small babies do experience orgasms. If asked, a mother may not have realized that the quivering of her infant was a convulsion of sheer joy. More likely than not it frightened her. Some mothers fear that the baby is having an epileptic seizure; others imagine that he is having a distressing dream of intrauterine life. Still other mothers think that the baby is suffering a partial loss of equilibrium, or fear of falling. But experienced observers now know that this tremor, or convulsion, under the pleasurable stimulation of mouth–breast contact or other pleasurable stimulation, is the orgasm reflex in its early form. You too as you nestled next to your mother, sucking from her breast, may have enjoyed an upsurge of good feeling so great that you not only exhibited the orgasm reflex, but you may well have experienced orgasm, though of course you do not remember it now.

A mother who enjoys her baby's pleasure as well as her own bodily sensations while nursing, is giving him one of his first positive introductions to sex. She is laying a healthy ground work for his later acceptance of his sexual self.

In the past, parents have also tended to think of the orgasm as being reserved for married adults, but they were wrong. Orgasms take place at every age and stage of life: in the very young and the very old, in the unmarried and the married, in men and in women; but at very different levels of intensity. In other words, it is natural and normal to all. One reason that adults have thought of orgasm as being strictly for the married person is that they confused the whole wonderful world of ecstatic feeling with one very specific function of the sexual act, namely, the begetting of babies. They forgot, or perhaps they never knew, that the orgasm reflex in varying levels of intensity belongs to everybody, whether one is in love or not, grown up or not, married or not, and need not be linked with procreation. (We are talking now not about intercourse but about orgasm.)

Let's return to the infant who put his thumb in his mouth and found it pure delight. If no grownup took his thumb away or otherwise made it impossible for him to reach his mouth, he probably felt most pleased with himself and with the sensations he experienced. Some parents have been taught to prohibit their infants from sucking on the ground that it isn't sanitary or that it might cause malformation of the teeth. Both of these beliefs are largely mistaken. If a baby gets the idea, even though unspoken, that sucking is not allowed or that it displeases his parents, he may not only turn to nail-biting later, but he may hanker after mouth activities all his life whenever he feels anxious or nervous or in special need of love. Some American psychologists feel that an excessive need to smoke may be attributed in part to lack of adequate sucking experience in infancy.

Now let us look at another aspect of developing sexuality. It may surprise you to learn that all babies discover very early that the process of excretion is a pleasurable experience. Nearly every mother has, at one time or another, found her darling cooing delightedly while playing with his own excrement. Some mothers can appreciate such a show of infantile pleasure, recognizing it for what it is. But others are repelled and as they clean the baby, they do so with such a briskness of hand touch that their displeasure is communicated to the baby. Sometimes such a woman can be heard to say, "What a dirty little baby you are!" in tones of disgust, and later when she has tidied him neatly she says, "Now you are my nice little fellow." A baby would have to be an idiot not to get the message, even though he does not consciously understand the words.

The nonverbal communication is, "What you produce from your body is somehow unlovable and undesirable." This is the beginning of sex shame, for the part of the body that relates most specifically to sex pleasure is also closely located anatomically to the anus. Thus most children become confused. They think that if mama doesn't like the anus or the urethra and what comes from them, she doesn't like the penis or the vagina either. In a little child's mind the difference is not yet clear.

About this time, furthermore, another important discovery is made by all intelligent babies. They discover their genitals. A little boy finds out that he has a penis and that it feels very pleasurable to touch; and a little girl discovers that she has a clitoris, which also feels pleasurable to touch. Usually such discoveries are made as early as a child locates and finds meaning in different parts of his body.

Unless his mother or his father are frightened by his discovery, he reaches for this delightful part of himself again and again, and it pleases him. He feels comforted. At first the reaching movements of the baby are random and accidental. But soon an intelligent child learns to be more direct and purposeful. Just as he discovers how to put his thumb in his mouth for comfort and for pleasure, he now learns to find his own genitals for the same reasons.

If at this time his mother communicates (nonverbally, of course, by her smiling acquiescence) that this activity is all right with her, he will enjoy untroubled pleasure in his own early sexuality. In fact he will, as I noted before, accept it as the good experience which, indeed, it is.

But if his parents give him the idea that "playing with himself" is bad or shameful, he will in all likelihood do one of two things, both of which are harmful to the development of healthy sexuality. Either he will learn to block off his sexual feeling (unconsciously, of course), or he will learn to enjoy sexual feelings in secret. Later he learns to feel guilty about forbidden activity, just as a punished puppy does who is caught making a puddle in the middle of the living-room rug.

Both reactions are detrimental for his future enjoyment of

healthy, adult sexuality in marriage. A little child's early discovery of sexuality and the pleasure of sexuality needs to be affirmed positively. Later he may need to be told when, where, how – but seldom, "don't".

Thus far we have seen that all the natural functions of the human body are pleasurable: breathing, sucking, eliminating, playing with the genitals, and body contact. Furthermore, the baby not only feels good physically, but feels he is a good person when he experiences them. If, however, he has been made to feel ashamed about acts which were meant to leave him with good feelings, he gets the wrong notion that when something is pleasurable, it must be evil, and that therefore he is a bad person.

Those of us who have been so conditioned have a lot of unlearning to do before we can enjoy healthy sexuality. We have to learn to trust our own healthy body feelings as being essentially good for us.

This brings us to the matter of feelings and emotion.

By definition, emotion is feeling in movement. Since we do not live solely in our minds but also in our whole body, and since our musculature is that part of us which is responsible for body movement, you will immediately see the relationship of the muscles to the expression of *any* feeling. For example, you discover that when you are angry you want to kick, bite, punch, scratch, scream, or throw; or perhaps all of them together. In other words, the large muscles that effect aggressive action of the kind just mentioned want to go into action.

If you feel sad the muscles that effect crying or sobbing are those that tense for action. If you are frightened the muscles that make it possible to scream or run go into action. If you are tenderly drawn to someone or something, the muscles of "reach" are activated.

Now if no one tells you that it is wrong to let your body move in these primary ways, you tend to move just as I have described. If the desirable primary movement causes no harm to anything or anyone, it is beneficial. But too often we forget to think before we act and harm results. Thus because parents are afraid of the potential destructiveness of primary expression of feeling, they tend to do something still more destructive. They tell their children, "Don't feel" – or at least, "Don't express your feelings."

What they actually say is, "Nice little girls don't get angry"; or, "Big, brave boys don't cry"; or, "Don't touch your penis; nice children don't do such things" – and so on and so on. They have sought to educate by a "don't" instead of by a "how". Most parents want to teach a child control, but many end up teaching him repression instead.

There is a vital difference between repression and control. Repression occurs when you try to deny a feeling and thus to stop its movement by tightening the muscles involved in its expression, just as a rider pulls frantically and almost uselessly on the reins of a runaway horse. Control, on the other hand, is learning how to express your feelings so that you have constructive results from your expression. You end up feeling satisfied and free of tension.

If tension builds sufficiently without release, it tends to go out of control. For example, let's suppose that someone hurts you. You feel like doubling up your fists and poking him in the nose, but you know that this will only lead to further trouble, so you find yourself simply doubling your fists and hanging on hard to your shoulder muscles that just ache to strike out.

Now, let's suppose that instead of suffering such tension you bring your fist down hard on the sofa. In this way you release your body tensions, no one gets hurt, and then a very interesting further thing happens. You become relaxed enough to *think*. Most of our problems today are solved by brain, not brawn. We are no longer like primitive men whose very lives depended on the speedy use of brawn in time of danger.

But our muscles still crave to go into action and we do have to relieve tension or we run the risk of either exploding or imploding. One of my friends made a very wise observation when he said, "If I inhibit the expression of my feelings, I store up tension to the point where I either explode or implode. If I explode, the cops get me. If I implode, the doctors get me. Now, what is a reasonable man to do?" This is one of the most intelligent ques-

HOW SEXUALITY DEVELOPS

tions that a civilized man could ask himself. What is a reasonable man to do with feelings which *must* move with out subjecting himself to the penalties of "explosion" or "implosion?"

There are many answers; active sports, for example, have helped a great many persons to "work off" excess adrenalin. It would be well if there were a lunging bag in every home and a thick foam rubber pad on every desk upon which fists could come down hard in times of exasperation. (A lunging bag moves slowly, quite unlike a punching bag which is likely to hit you in the nose and make you angrier than ever.)

You have the key to *freedom from tension* if you remember that the goal is controlled expression of your emotions – not repression of them. First you acknowledge what you *do* feel and then you let this feeling move in satisfying and constructive ways. Recognize, for example, that you do want to cry, or you do want to curl up in someone's arms, or you do want to reach out for comfort and love, or that you do want to strike out in anger. Next ask yourself how you can do these things without ill effects.

Could you, for example, cry in the arms of some trusted human being without being called a crybaby? Lacking such a person, could you cry in your own room? What greater friend could there be than one who has sense enough, when he sees your sadness, to say to you, "Have a good cry, dear, it will make you feel better", as indeed it does.

Thus the *expression* of feeling relieves tension and in turn frees your brain for the job of problem solving, which is what brains are for. Often your thought processes are paralysed by fear that you will "get out of control".

About now you may be asking, "What has all this to do with sex and my sexual development?"

It has a great deal to do with sex – more than you might suspect. For example, the tender emotion of love, expressed sexually, cannot move through the muscular blockade of repressed anger. If by any chance it tries to break through, it comes out hard like a hammer blow instead of gently, warmly, caressingly. A partner exposed to such "loving" can only withdraw instead of respond. Then the "lover" feels rejected. In rejection his anger is increased rather than diminished. Shakespeare said it so well when he wrote, "Hell hath no fury like a woman scorned."

If our hypothetical lover could recognize that he is carrying his repressed anger into a lovemaking situation, he might find a way to get rid of it before so much as touching his girl. I can guarantee that she will respond to him more affirmatively if he does so.

Many persons, even young persons, have so armoured themselves against recognizing their own feelings that they have lost the ability to sense feelings in others. They are embarrassed in the presence of feeling. They say that they would feel silly if they cried, or acknowledged fear, or reached out tenderly. Actually, they are afraid of what might happen if they let go.

To understand the extent of this fear, however, you must also recognize that no person braces himself against these feelings unless at some time in the past, he learned he had to do so in order to get what he needed for survival. His very life depended on his mother's approval – or so it seemed to him at the time. So as a kind of life or death measure, he learned to stop expressing those feelings because such expression brought him disapproval.

Now, of course, as a young adult, his habit of resisting the expression of emotions remains. It has become chronic. And even though that which inhibited him as an infant no longer is a cause of inhibition, his habit of blocking feelings goes on and he tends to think that his frozen unexpressiveness is just the way he is.

However, you must remember that *no one* is born immobile or unexpressive. People get that way because they have been punished for emotional mobility, because someone on whom they were dependent for life itself would not tolerate such evidences of strong emotion.

Let's go back now to other aspects of sexual development.

First the baby enjoyed suckling. A little later he found pleasure in fondling his own genitals. Some children have a few other sexual experiences as they grow up. For example, a child is curious and if he has an opportunity to live intimately with another child (a sister, a brother, a cousin), he and that other child may have experimented with each other. Most often, the experimentation among children takes the form of satisfying curiosity about differences in anatomy. Almost any nursery-school teacher can tell you of the countless times she has chanced on a little boy and girl undressing each other just to see how the other is made. This is perfectly harmless and almost all enterprising children try it at least once. Some youngsters, having discovered how good it feels to touch their own genital organs, wonder if it will feel as pleasant to have someone else touch them; or they want to see if their friend is as pleasured as they are by the experience. All this is a very innocent and natural part of growing up. However, just as some adults are afraid of childhood masturbation, so some are afraid of experimental sex play between young children. Yet in almost all instances such play is a regular and normal part of growing into adulthood and no harm comes from it.

CHAPTER 2

Noncoital sex

ONE of the big problems that you, the unmarried, face is how you will handle your sexual urges in those long years which seem to stretch out forever before that walk down the aisle becomes feasible.

One way is through masturbation. This perfectly good act does not carry a good name. The word stems from two Latin words, *manus* and *stupro*, meaning to pollute with the hand. Now, of all the silly ideas that anyone could get, this is one of the silliest, for obviously the genital organs are not polluted by caressing them with one's hands. Let me affirm again: This can be a healthy and normal way to enjoy sexual feeling when you are not ready or able to share loving sexuality with a person of the opposite sex. A better name for masturbation is autoeroticism, or self-gratification.

In the past, parents were afraid that if a baby discovered how pleasant it was to touch his genitals, he wouldn't want to do much of anything else. Also, and more important, parents were worried that later on in adolescence if boys and girls played with each other's genitals, they would be led into the act of intercourse and thus expose themselves to the possibility of having a baby long before they were ready to marry and care for children. So adults acquired the mistaken notion that it was wrong for children to touch and enjoy their genitals at all.

An incredible number of old wives' tales have grown up about this matter of masturbation. In my day we were told that we would go crazy if we did it. Of course, this is nonsense. No one ever went crazy from masturbating though a lot of people have been crazed from fear and guilt about doing something that they had been told was wrong.

A more modern myth is that it is all right to masturbate if you don't do it too much. But this sets up almost as much anxiety as some of the horrendous older tales, since no one tells you how much is too much. The truth is that autoeroticism is self-determining, like eating, indulging in a sport, or any other natural function. If you overeat, for example, you have a distended, uncomfortable feeling in your stomach. If you overmasturbate you will feel uncomfortable in your genital area. Nothing more, nothing less – as simple as that.

Another more recent myth is that people who masturbate will not enjoy sex in marriage as much as those who don't. Scientific research shows quite the opposite. Young persons who have developed their sexual feeling and their ability to come to orgasm through masturbatory techniques, have a better chance to enjoy fully satisfying sexuality in marriage. The truth is that all people can and do feel gratified when their genital organs are pleasurably stimulated, as long as they are not frightened about these good body feelings by unnecessary guilt which may have been instilled in them by well-meaning but ill-informed adults.

I might say right here that the positive values of masturbation are not limited to the young and unmarried, though autoeroticism serves a particularly useful function for you – the young adult. In addition to releasing sexual tensions which can become enormously troubling at this time, it is Nature's way of preparing you for the later enjoyment of sexuality with a partner. It also protects young people from leaping into sexual experiences with partners whom they do not love just to satisfy their sexual needs.

One very faulty notion that people in the past had was that young adults could walk into marriage sexually mature, with no practice and no skill, and then become sexual artists simply through a bungling sort of experimentation or by reading a book or two. Their ignorance masqueraded as "innocence" or "purity", but it was ignorance just the same, and if you look around you at the divorce statistics and then note that sex ignorance is one of the important causes for those statistics, you will know that this idea is erroneous indeed.

Adults who developed their sexual awareness and responses as they were growing up are shown to have a much better chance of continuing that growth successfully in marriage than those who denied the existence or the expression of their sexual feelings. Let me repeat: A person who has learned how to come to orgasm through masturbation is much more likely to be a good sex partner in marriage than one who has not. After all, learning how to move sexually is not unlike learning to dance. Generally, an individual has to practise the steps by himself before he can move sensitively with another in dancing. If he stumbles and shuffles along and has no sense of rhythm, he will not be a very welcome dance partner. At best, even after he can dance quite well by himself, it may still take some skilled coaching to help him adjust his dance synchronously with that of another.

If you have already discovered the pleasure of self-gratification, you will have discovered a number of very fascinating things about yourself when you are sexually stimulated. First, you will find that your breathing quickens, that your face may become flushed, and that your whole body seems to want to move rhythmically. Presently, as you reach a peak of excitement, there comes a quivering, involuntary, convulsive-like movement which is the orgasm described earlier.

As you repeat this experience over the years, you will find that you have developed a characteristic way of bringing yourself to climax (orgasm) that is unique to you.

Some girls, for example, discover that their greatest pleasure comes from rhythmically moving the clitoris through traction of some sort. Others by pressing and releasing their legs; others by a circular movement of their fingers over the pubic area and along the sides of the clitoris. Some discover that they get more pleasurable sensation by stroking themselves very hard or very fast; others by doing so slowly and gently.

Boys develop their own unique patterns also. A few masturbate by pressing the penis upon a bed, and then rocking back and forth in a movement not unlike that used in intercourse. More frequently, a boy uses some sort of back and forth movement of his hand around the shank of his penis. Some boys learn to postpone the ejaculation for as long as possible for its pleasurable potential. Others train themselves to "come" very fast, mostly to avoid possible discovery by adults who might censure them. (One of the few negative aspects of masturbation is this learning to do it too fast.)

Later on, in marriage, a man will be at an advantage in making love to his wife if he has learned to be slow and leisurely in coming to orgasm, for the average woman takes much longer to arrive at climax than the average man (though there is good reason to believe that this is due to inhibition because of cultural influence rather than to her nature as a female).

Boys usually imagine themselves in all sorts of erotic encounters with girls, and vice versa. Usually the fantasies of boys involve the viewing of a nude or seminude girl (or girls) who may, or may not, be making love.

A girl's fantasies are more likely to be about a strong male overpowering her with his seductive persuasiveness. She is rarely aroused by imagined male nudity, but *is* excited by a male show of strength and purposefulness or male admiration of her.

Sometimes boys associate an object with sexual arousal. For example, a boy may have experienced his first conscious sexual pleasure in erection when, as a tiny child, he was lying on the floor looking up at his mother. What he may have seen as he lay there was her pink underpanties atop a pair of legs. Later he discovers that if he imagines the pink underpanties he can, and will, get an erection. Later still, in adult lovemaking, he may desire that this *object* be present when he makes love to his wife. Such a desire is called *fetishistic*, and the object is called a *fetish*. It is nothing to worry about, for as a boy's experience in lovemaking grows, he can learn to enlarge the range of stimuli that can affect his developing sexuality.

Girls also have something that resembles fetishistic behaviour, but it is not called that, since it is rare that they attach sexual feeling to an object for self-stimulation. However, they do have fantasies which serve as sexual stimulants just the same, and sometimes girls become quite dependent upon these. For example, many a girl is excited by a spanking fantasy, even though she wouldn't want to act it out for love nor money. Such a fantasy is easy to understand, for a little girl who has been spanked experiences, as an aftermath of the pain, a rosy glow of sexual excitation in the same general anatomical area as her sexual organs. As a child she hated the spanking with its humiliation and discomfort, but she also liked the resulting aftersensation. Sometimes parents have been heard to remark, "Our child seems to be asking for a spanking." This could be true, you know. But it is also one good reason for not spanking children, at least not on the bottom, for who wants to use pain as a stimulus for pleasure?

There are literally thousands of fantasies. No matter how bizarre they are, they should not become worries, since they are practically never acted upon, except by mutual agreement between partners who think that a given fantasy might be fun to try out. A fantasy's chief function is to excite to a high pitch of sexuality quickly and intensely, and thus bypass a long, slow buildup of erotic feeling. An additional function is to enrich the sexual experience, for after all, a human being can carry himself on the magic carpet of imagination into any experience that he chooses. This is one way that men and women bring variety into their lovemaking, keeping it from growing boring.

Some people are afraid that they are being disloyal to their partners if they indulge in such fantasies. But they need not feel so. Almost all people do it and these sexual fantasies have nothing to do with disloyality. As I said before, they are merely additional sex stimulants and sex enrichers. No one in his right mind would desert a real partner for a fantasy, but a fantasy can sometimes make sex with a real partner more fun. And it is a lifesaver for the person who hasn't any partner at all.

This brings us to the whole matter of partners. I said earlier that one of the great functions of sex is to draw people together. Sexual feeling causes this to happen in a general way and also in a very specific way.

In the general way, it makes us enjoy being cuddled by our own parents. It makes us want to put our arms around a friend's shoulder. It even makes us want to pat our dogs or stroke our kittens.

In a specific way, it draws us to one special individual who is more attractive to us than any other. We find that we not only want to touch and be touched by this special person, but we want to share our whole personality with him (or her), and our lives as well. This is what we call love.

There can, of course, be sexual attraction without love, and we will talk of this later and also about how to differentiate the kind of love which is enduring from that which is infatuation.

No one knows exactly why one person attracts us more than another, although there are all sorts of theories on the subject. Some social scientists feel that if a boy has had a very good relationship with his mother he may be attracted to a girl who in some way resembles her; or if a girl has had a father whom she admires she is apt to be drawn to a boy who is like him; but it doesn't always work out that way.

Another hypothesis is that we seek those persons who are most like our dream images of a mate – the fairy tale "dream prince or princess" that we have carried deep within us from childhood.

An opinion often advanced by marriage guidance counsellors is that we are drawn to those who satisfy our unconscious needs. An unconscious need is simply a longing that we carried over from childhood – some experience that we needed then but didn't have. The satisfaction of such needs is so vital that the adult still strives unconsciously for its fulfilment. If a person comes along who understands, accepts, and satisfies those longings in a constructive way, the deprived individual is not only helped into more and more adult forms of loving, but is overwhelmingly drawn to that person.

There are many other ideas about sexual attraction, some quite interesting. But for now let us simply accept the fact that this mysterious something called attraction does exist and that it operates on a highly selective basis. This means that while one person may not in the least cause your heart to beat faster, another will draw you to him as a bee is drawn to the opening clover. Gradually, after many experiments with attraction, you will learn what kind of person goes on being interesting to you long after the initial period of infatuation has passed. Just remember that almost all human relationships begin with the magnetic force of sex in some form, but those which endure must have something more.

Somewhere along the way, a boy gets more and more interested in one special girl, or a girl in one special boy. This can happen at any age, but rather regularly it begins to happen in the mid and late teens. About then many boys and girls begin to "go steady".

This practice is nothing more or less than an experiment in the permanent pairing that will come later in marriage. It is a chance to try, in temporary form, what being closely linked with another person may be like. Many adults advise teenagers not to go steady, because they feel that a boy and girl may get so involved with each other at so young an age that they won't give themselves a chance to know any others.

Older people realize that if the young couple's relationship culminates in marriage before the boy and girl are mature, they may eventually find that they have made a poor choice. It is true that teenagers do change tremendously, sometimes almost perceptibly from month to month until they reach their early twenties. Ask any man of twenty-one. He will tell you that he would hardly recognize the boy he was at sixteen.

If you should get so involved with one girl at sixteen that you don't even look at any other girl, you may miss your chance for finding the kind of woman to whom you are most attracted and with whom you feel at home. You need a broad base for choice, just as you need to see a lot of the world before choosing which part of it you want to spend your life in; or, as you need to expose yourself to many occupational experiences before choosing a life-long vocation.

Let us acknowledge that a young adult is sometimes lucky and finds the permanent choice of mate in the very first partner he falls in love with, but these are the rare ones. However, most young persons like to go steady just the same, for they feel that this is one way that they can get to know one person well.

As boys and girls grow closer they usually want to be affectionate with each other. Here again is the sexual urge at work. They may want to hug and kiss and caress, and if the relationship deepens, they may want very much to touch and be touched by each other genitally. This is generally called petting.

Many times young people make the mistake of *arousing* each other sexually through petting, but *not satisfying* each other. This can lead at times to negative tension. Firstly, it stimulates urges that may become unbearable. Sometimes a young couple may marry prematurely just to relieve the tension, though they may not be the best partners for each other.

Secondly, the boy may suffer real pain unless he relieves himself through masturbation soon after such a petting session. Pelvic congestion in the girl is equally bad.

Thirdly, the girl can, by such petting techniques, be badly conditioned to switch on the red stoplight just when she is getting sexually aroused, so that later in marriage, when she *wants* a green light all the way, she finds that she is unable to move on into orgastic release. All in all, petting *without* orgastic release is bad business. If two teenagers do decide to pet, they would be wise to see to it that each comes to orgasm.

Mind you, I am not saying "have intercourse". I am talking about something else – namely, *noncoital* orgasm. Noncoital orgasm means sexual satisfaction and release without intercourse. This practice is as old as mankind. Good lovers from time immemorial have found numerous ways to bring each other to climax without recourse to penile penetration as in intercourse. Mutual caressing of the genitals is one noncoital form of sexual activity. If you ask any sophisticated married man or woman if such an activity is pleasurable, he or she will tell you that it can be every bit as satisfying as intercourse itself. Many women, particularly, find it more satisfying. Actually, a man's hands and fingers (as also a woman's) can be more skilful in the range of stimulating activity that they can perform than are the genital organs themselves.

Here again, adults have been so afraid that the young would engage in intercourse and thus risk an unwanted pregnancy that they have categorically negated all forms of sexual fulfilment until the necessary social safeguards for the begetting of a child were met, namely marriage.

It is time to reconsider and to overcome this fear. Teenagers learn to drive cars. A car is a dangerous machine in the hands of an untrained, untaught, immature, and undisciplined person. Factually, auto accidents occur more frequently than sex accidents. But a well-taught, well-disciplined person handles a car with responsibility and safety largely because he has graduated successfully from a driver education course. Parents see to it that he gets such a course. They don't say, "No driving until you are twenty-one." They do say, "Pass the course and then you can drive."

So it may be with sex in the future. There may come a day when parents will not say, "No sex", but will say, "Learn how to express sexuality safely and responsibly so that it may bring satisfaction to you and to your partner without casualty to anyone."

Thus mutual petting to orgasm by partners who love, respect, and care for each other's well-being, and who have learned how to direct their impulses so that they experience orgasm but do not expose themselves to the creation of a child, may be one step on the road to sexual maturity – one form of sexual expression for the young person who, in general, may not yet be ready for the full responsibility or implications of intercourse, but who is ready to share his love sexually with a partner.

Married lovers often call such petting "foreplay" because they end it with orgasm through intercourse; but it can just as easily end in orgasm for both partners without intercourse and it can be just as satisfying. *In such foreplay lies the art of sex.*

Petting, if it is to be fully rewarding, must be a natural outgrowth of love. If it is not, if it is only indulged in "for kicks", it tends to have little significance other than momentary pleasurable sensation. However, when petting is a genuine reaching out of one human being to another whom he loves, all manifestations of that love take on a significant and long-remembered character. Precious experiences sink deeply into memory and blessedly bathe one's consciousness for years thereafter.

An atmosphere of approval is necessary for any two people to feel loving. Many times young wives tell me that their husbands will criticize them one moment and then to make love the next. The fact is that a criticized person doesn't feel like making love. All of us need to know that the persons to whom we expose our bodies and our souls, as it were, like and approve of us.

I suppose that there are very few of us who haven't felt squeamish or unhappy about some aspects of our own bodies. Therefore, we need to have a beloved person tell us that we are beautiful, that our skin is nice, that our eyes sparkle, that our limbs feel smooth to touch, that we smell sweet.

We could also learn a thing or two from the Europeans who teach all boys and girls to use a bidet regularly. A bidet is a kind of washbasin which you sit in and thoroughly wash your genital organs. Girls need to push back the foreskin covering the clitoris, just as boys need to push back the foreskin covering the penis (if they are uncircumcized), and thoroughly wash. Otherwise, the foreskin sticks to the clitoris (or to the penis) and causes adhesions, as well as unpleasant odours.

Most girls and boys like to be touched gently, approvingly, warmly, but if one or the other is tense to begin with and just can't relax, he may need the other to help him to relax emotionally, which does, of course, result in physical relaxation.

This is why I discussed so extensively in the previous chapter the importance of resolving those muscular blocks created by repressed anger, or sadness, or fear, before trying to express love. Often a word of praise will be enough to accomplish this. It is worth the try. People vary in their responses to different stimuli. Adult lovers must learn the response patterns of their beloveds. Young people, if they are to learn how to be successful lovers, must do likewise. One woman, for example, may be "turned on" by breast contact; another by gentle caressing of the nape of her neck; another by kissing, another by direct genital play; and most by honest praise and approval.

All the surfaces of the skin have nerve endings that report pleasure to the brain, but certain areas of the body contain large concentrations of such nerve endings, namely, the breast, the lips, the mouth, the clitoris (in the girl), the penis (in the boy), the anus and the buttocks and the lower back.

The penis is most sensitively pleasure-giving around the corona (the enlarged area near the tip); the clitoris is most pleasure-giving in the area directly around and above it but not directly on it, for it is too sensitive for much friction. The back of the vaginal opening is also rich in such nerve endings.

If a girl wishes to please her beloved she needs to learn how to handle his penis with skill and reverence just as a boy needs to learn how to handle a girl's clitoral area with skill and tenderness.

No two girls, for example, will masturbate exactly alike, nor will any two girls require exactly the same kind of caressing of their genitals to bring them to orgasm. The same statement could be made for boys. When married people seek help in coming to orgasm, it is often suggested that each partner show the other exactly, with his or her own hand, what pattern of caress is most likely to produce a climax (orgasm). Many married couples are embarrassed to do this because they have been made to feel ashamed to acknowledge that they touch themselves when they are alone. What a pity, because this is one very helpful way to become skilful in sexual expression.

It is a pity also that so many girls have been made afraid of the penis. Once upon a time, in more ancient cultures, the penis was worshipped as an object of great beauty and as a symbol of fertility. In the Far East today one can still find carved penises which are sold as art objects. In India the act of lovemaking was considered an act fit for the gods and there are temples glorifying the gods in all sorts of postures of love. It is hard in Western art to find beautiful male figures with an erect penis, though the female figure is glorified at every hand.

Both male and female bodies, however, can be beautiful. The

sooner one learns to think of the genitalia of both sexes as beautiful parts of bodies, attractive and appealing, and worthy of the most tender and expert handling, the better the lovemaking will be.

Both male and female secrete a lubricating fluid under sexual excitation. This is quite essential to the woman if sexual contact is to be comfortable. A dry hand on a dry clitoris can be painful rather than pleasurable. If Nature has not quite caught up with a girl's sexual needs, experienced lovers use some other form of lubricant, such as saliva, or cold cream, or vaseline. With such aids a natural flow of lubrication soon takes over its pleasure-giving role.

Lovemaking needs a safe place, an environment that is protected from all intrusion. I might say that it needs protection from inner pricklings of guilt as well. This is one of the reasons why teenage lovemaking often turns out to be so unsatisfactory for both partners, but especially for the girl. (Boys, from long solitary practice in masturbation, have usually learned to snatch a bit of momentary pleasure, whenever or wherever, even if they feel guilty about it.) When it comes to sharing love feelings with a girl, boys may be just as inept as girls for this takes *time* and *safety*, careful planning, *artistry* and freedom from guilt.

One's own home, with affirmation and consent from parents, would ideally be the best place for the expression of intimate love. A parked car is one of the worst. Wherever the element of apprehensiveness enters, positive feelings tend to disappear.

When I have asked boys what they value most in girls, the answer is almost invariably, "responsiveness". I believe that women are equally concerned with responsiveness in the men they care for. No one likes to expose his intimate feelings of love to a cold or rigid partner, but a mobile, responsive, loving person is irresistible.

Birth control is the subject of a later chapter, but even at this point it is well to say that if the partners are not using a safe birth control method, a boy should take great care not to ejaculate anywhere near the entrance to the girl's vagina to avoid the risk of pregnancy for the girl. Even though she has an intact hymen and has not had intercourse, there is a natural opening in the hymen through which menstruation occurs. If a boy ejaculates near this opening, sperm may find their way into the vagina and cause pregnancy even though the girl remains technically a virgin.

CHAPTER 3

Premarital intercourse – pro and con

THE most frequent question asked by college students is: "How do you rid yourself of guilt and shame so that you can enjoy sex at all, even after you're married – let alone before?"

This is a tough problem, for the roots of guilt are very deep. However, many adults even in our time believe that if they tell youth that sex is good, but only *in* marriage, all will be well; they hope that when marriage comes along, the old taboos and fears will vanish, and healthy young people will be able at last to enjoy their sexuality.

The trouble is, it doesn't always work that way. You can't be conditioned for twenty-odd years to eschew sex – indeed, to believe that it is immoral except in marriage – and then, with the utterance of a marriage vow, expect the effect of such conditioning to disappear into thin air.

To a greater or lesser degree most of you reading this book are victims of unintentional negative sex conditioning. Whatever sexuality you *have* enjoyed has more than likely been partly spoiled by a nagging sense that you ought not to be enjoying it.

To do parents justice, they don't intend that their preaching shall have this effect on you. What they think they are doing is protecting you from sexual casualties. However, in the process they teach you fear. Of course, *they* were taught fear, and fear tends to beget fear.

If I could wish for every youth the best possible approach to sex, I would wish him a set of parents whose own sex lives were wonderful and who could fearlessly affirm the healthy sexuality of their children. But you must realize that because of their crippling indoctrination many of the parents of your generation have never known sexual ecstasy. A great many of the women have never even experienced orgasm. How could they be other than frightened about sex?

Furthermore, you must understand that the demon Envy can cause some adults to create sexual fear in youth. Graham Greene wrote in his novel *End of the Affair*: "When you are miserable, you envy other people's happiness."

Envy, as all of us know, is a most harmful force, for when we envy, we tend to become very nasty and destructive of everything other people enjoy.

Wilhelm Reich called the neurotic need of sexually unhappy people to destroy the sexual happiness of others *the emotional plague*, and plague it is indeed.

You will have to learn to recognize emotionally plagued people and avoid absorption of their fears; otherwise you may be hurt.

Don't expose whatever tenderness, healing, and blessedness you have found in sex to sex-negative people. Expressions of love are your own special treasures, to be shared only with those who know how to love and who are not corroded by hate and fear.

This problem of whom to confide in presents a great dilemma, for when you are in love you want to shout it from the housetops.

You also genuinely need the advice and assistance which a mature and *sex-positive* adult can give. How are you going to find such a trustworthy person?

If your own parents have been frank with you all along in their answers to the sex questions you have put to them, and especially *if* they seem to love each other, and *if* they have treated with respect the members of the opposite sex whom you have brought to your home, then *they* may be the best of all persons to talk with.

Among professionals, those best trained in sex and love affairs are the marriage guidance counsellors who, by the way, are just as concerned with the problems of unmarried lovers as they are with those of married couples. Doctors and clergymen who have been trained in sex education may also be helpful.

You can count on them to advise you responsibly in the many

technicalities with which you should be acquainted if you are going to achieve love and a healthy sexuality.

It helps in dissipating guilt if you realize that many of the religious precepts denying sex pleasure to the unmarried are based on conditions which existed at a time long in the past. Their continuance into the present is superstition and reflects not only ignorance of scientific technology but faulty knowledge of the social psychology of today.

For example, it was once thought that all men preferred virgins and that any girl not a virgin at the time of marriage was "damaged goods" and likely to be rejected.

Today we know that most intelligent men consider virginity immaterial. It is about as useful in a prospective wife as an appendix. What counts most is a wife's ability to respond warmly, and to have developed the many other human skills which make her interesting and creative. How can she be such a woman if she hasn't been growing toward it in her girlhood?

To the girl or the boy who is struggling unnecessarily with the spectre of guilt, I suggest the following: Ask yourself:

(1) Is what I feel and express honest? Does it leave me feeling good about myself? Does it do likewise for my partner?

(2) Do I fully trust the person to whom I am expressing my love sexually? (Sexuality must be rooted in personal trust, for nowhere else are we more exposed or more vulnerable.)

(3) Does my sexual activity harm anyone?

(4) Does my sexual activity involve risks I cannot handle?

If the answers are Yes to questions (1) and (2) and No to questions (3) and (4), then I suggest the following to reinforce your conviction that the relationship is good: *Read* to enlarge your vision. Discover that there is no straight and narrow path to heaven, but rather that heaven is reached in many ways. For example, read some anthropology, like Bronislaw Malinowski's *Sexual Life of Savages in North-Western Melanesia*. Read a great love story like D. H. Lawrence's 'The Man who died'. Read some historical accounts of sexual customs such as *Sexual Pleasure in*

Marriage by Jerome and Julia Rainer. You might look at the remarkable illustrations in some of the new art books, particularly those depicting the erotic art of various historical periods, or read some of the work of the modern psychologist-sexologists, like Albert Ellis's *Art and Practice of Love*, or Edward and Ruth Brecher's *Analysis of Human Sexual Response*, or *Living With Sex: The Student's Dilemma* by Richard F. Hettlinger.

Next, learn to trust your own observation. Judge things by the good or bad effect they have upon you and upon those with whom you are in contact.

If your sexual activity seems to make you a nicer person to live with generally, if it increases your interest in life, in work, in study, in growth, you may trust your own conclusion that it is good for you. On the other hand, if you are miserable afterwards, you must ask yourself if something is wrong with the sexuality itself or with this particular relationship – and see what you can do to improve the situation.

Almost every young person feels like a cheat when he or she engages in sexual activity with a lover while knowing that his parents, if apprised of it, would not only disapprove but would withdraw all moral and economic support. Such absolute disapproval puts a boy or girl in a terrible dilemma.

A college student, for example, knows that he must have his parents' support if he is to continue his education; yet often his whole being, rational and emotional, also tells him that he must express his love. What is he to do?

Fortunately for youth, the day is fast coming when such absolute stands will not be taken by parents.

In the meantime, many thousands of young people decide, in their dilemma, to deceive their parents. They keep silent even about something as important as their love lives; thus parents and youth are shut off from each other in a crucial area which should be blessed by openness. Ninety-five per cent of the dangers of premarital sex could be eliminated if parents would make their homes and their own knowledge available to their children as they would in all other areas of life.

Perhaps you may be able to persuade your parents to do this if you approach them rationally and honestly. Ask them to reflect on what the world might be like, for example, if a boy had to use a neighbour's car to teach himself to drive, in some dark alley without benefit of parental advice and approval. Yet this is just the way many parents behave about sex.

One aspect of guilt I haven't mentioned at all occurs when a girl (and usually it is the girl) discovers that she has made a wrong choice of partner – that she has lavished love and trust on someone who has simply exploited her for selfish sexual reasons.

Girls need to know, I think, that some boys – far more than girls – may want sex for sex's sake and not as an expression of personal affection, and will use any ruse to get it.

If a girl has misjudged a boy's true feelings and has intercourse with him before she has known him in other ways which could test the nature of his love for her, she runs the risk of discovering that sex, not love, has motivated this boy. She may feel tricked or abandoned, and swamped by negative emotions. She may also be overwhelmed with guilt. All the old wives' tales about "loose women" may torture her, and she may look upon herself as a sorry creature indeed.

The only real mistake this girl has made is that of misjudging character, not in expressing her sexuality. She must learn more about the nature of boys in general, and the nature of *the* boy in particular with whom she chooses to share sexuality.

Remember once again, all love contains sex – but not all sex springs from love. Let the love be manifest first and let the sex follow if you would not run the risk of losing your self-respect.

In the final analysis, we all have to grow up sufficiently to decide for ourselves what we deserve to feel guilty about (and to make up for our sins as best we can). But we must differentiate real guilty from false or induced guilt. The latter must be discarded. In other words, we have to become ready to take the responsibility for our own acts. A college professor of mine once gave me his definition of maturity: "You are mature when you become your own mother and your own father and stand ready to yield your self up to the full hazards of independence."

Quite an assignment!

As you yourself decide whether – or when – your sexual activity will include intercourse, there are other factors besides the resolution of guilt to consider.

First is the matter of physical and psychic readiness.

Many boys from about fifteen years of age on are bursting to experience intercourse because they have been told that this is the only "real" form of sexual expression. It isn't, of course, but the folklore persists nevertheless.

On the other hand, very few girls under seventeen or eighteen desire anything more than petting. This adds up to a real discrepancy in goals, and it also leads to the classic war-of-the-sexes game, which is rather unfortunate.

Too often a boy says to a girl, "If only you loved me you would go to bed with me", and the girl, needing love and affection desperately, acquiesces. However, if she has been sufficiently cherished by her family, particularly by her father, she may feel secure enough to say to the boy, "If only you loved *me* you wouldn't ask me to do something I am not ready for. After all, I'm the one who takes the risks."

Petting to orgasm is one resolution of this dilemma (see Chapter 2), for not only is it satisfying to both partners but it carries none of the attendant risks of intercourse and is usually much more welcomed by the girl at her level of sexual development.

But let's look at what can happen to the boy who *insists* on intercourse:

(1) He can have it with a prostitute.

This is usually so unaesthetic and so without love that it can result in his "tuning out" sex for a long time to come. Many boys acquire a cynical attitude about love and sex from such contacts. Dissociation of love from sex is unfortunate since sex at its best must have meaning and value. Also it must be remembered that prostitution is illegal, so when a boy resorts to this outlet he does so with a certain degree of shame and guilt which is not helpful to him in his total sexual development. It is often destructive of self-esteem to have to pay for that which should be given freely. Finally, it exposes him to venereal disease.

(2) He can *force* his girl to have intercourse with him.

I use the word force, for coercion of any kind is still force – even when it says, in essence, "I won't date you unless you have intercourse with me." A boy who resorts to such coercion will be less than satisfied with the result because any sex which results from coercive or exploitative methods generally leaves the exploiter the loser. He will find that intercourse was not what it was cracked up to be.

(3) A third possibility is that he can try to find a sympathetic and experienced older woman with whom he can establish a tender and loving sexual relationship.

A boy is probably lucky if he finds the rare older woman who sensitively introduces him to sex. One can appreciate the wisdom of the ancients who maintained temple priestesses for the education of their young men and temple priests for the education of their young women. However, the average American boy has little or no access to contemporary equivalents.

(4) This brings us to a fourth solution, and here we will hypothesize an unusual situation.

Let's suppose that a boy of sixteen has found a girl of sixteen whom he truly loves and whose parents are not unalterably against premarital intercourse. They have provided her with a safe place and with a thorough education in birth control. His own parents, as well as hers, are ready to back the two of them to the limit. Such a situation, you will agree, might exist, though rarely – perhaps only one time in a hundred – but let's look at it. Even here the ironic thing is that this girl might be the very one who would be likely to say, "I'm not quite ready for it myself." I have known of situations like that. When a girl isn't pressured by fear or loss of love, the chances are ten to one that she will prefer coming to orgasm by the petting route rather than by intercourse until she is seventeen or eighteen.

All right, what next? The boy and girl are now at college, or they will have found their first jobs. Perhaps they will already be economically independent; others will have a long road ahead before they can support themselves.

If intercourse is to be practicable at all for these young adults, they must be able to guarantee the following conditions:

(a) That they will not conceive an unwanted child.

(b) That, should they fail in their use of birth control methods, they will be able to handle the problem of an unplanned pregnancy.

(c) That they can provide an aesthetically satisfying environment for the flowering of their sexual love, such as a safe place for lovemaking without fear of interruptions or police intervention.

(d) They must be free from feelings of guilt. In other words, they must be able to tell themselves, with conviction, that what they are doing is in accord with what they believe to be right; otherwise, the sexual experience itself can be overshadowed by their fears.

I think you will have concluded by now that sexual intercourse involves adult responsibilities which few, if any, young teenagers can meet (especially those under sixteen), and which relatively few seventeen- or eighteen-year-olds can successfully meet without effective assistance from parents or other experienced adults. But by nineteen or twenty a considerable number are likely to become sufficiently mature and self-reliant.

Today many college administrators have decided that it is wiser to assist the college-age student who wants to lead a safe, sane, and educated sex life than to set prohibitions in his way. These prohibitions have always been broken and the casualties have been costly. Therefore, college medical officers on the whole now provide birth control advice for students who ask for it. Furthermore, many college staff members are prepared to offer students the equivalent of marriage counselling.

I know some parents now who have not only provided their daughters and their sons with a thorough grounding in birth control methods, but have supplied them with birth control equipment and definitive training in its use. Furthermore, and better yet, they have offered their unmarried children the sanctity and the safety of the home for the sexual expression of love.

Most of you, however, lacking such complete affirmation and

protection, will be happier with petting to orgasm than with taking on the additional burden of responsibility which goes with intercourse: especially as you learn that petting to orgasm can be fully satisfying, both physically and emotionally.

To sum up, intercourse is only one means of sexual enjoyment, and before you indulge in it, you ought to feel quite sure in your own mind that you realize fully what is involved, and that you love and trust your partner.

CHAPTER 4

The art of
first intercourse

LET us suppose that you are deeply in love, that you have established a relationship of trust with a partner and that you can meet the responsibilities inherent in coital activity. What then do you need to know about the art and science of intercourse?

Let's assume, to begin with, that you are or will be thoroughly educated in birth control methods. (See Chapter 5.)

Next, if you, the girl, are a virgin, then you, the boy, need to know how to effect first penetration so that she suffers little, if any discomfort. If the two of you have been petting to orgasm, as you may have been, you will have gone a long way toward stretching the hymen and preparing the passage for the penis. Actually, very few girls need have any fear that they will not be able to stretch to receive even the largest penis, for the vagina is considered "infinitely expandable". However, to a virgin, a penis can feel tremendous. If a boy takes time, over many days, to insert first one finger, then two, then a thumb, he will gradually effect the necessary stretching, so that when he is ready to enter, the girl will suffer a minimum of distress. She can also take responsibility for herself. She can learn to insert her own fingers into her vagina and gently stretch the opening.

Occasionally a hymen is so thick and resistant that it requires surgical intervention. If reasonable and patient stretching does not make it possible for the penis to enter without pain, a girl should consult a gynaecologist who will examine her and arrange to remove the hymen under local anaesthesia. No boy should attempt to break through a hymen of this sort by penile thrust, for the girl can be permanently traumatized so that future sex for her may become distasteful.

Lubrication is important, just as in loveplay. Dry abrasive contact of the sexual organs with any surface is painful. Saliva, cold cream, Noxzema – all are satisfactory lubricants. Of course, in most instances, Nature provides the perfect lubricant, once sexual excitation is sufficient. The only trouble is, that when the experience is new and the participants are a bit anxious, Nature may not be very generous with lubrication.

If a boy tries to effect entrance without it, a girl will in all likelihood pull away from him.

Slow, gentle pressure is better for the girl than an impatient thrust. If the girl controls both the depth and the speed of penetration, she will be more comfortable, for she can then decide how much she feels ready for. If she has been well loved and well stimulated before penetration is attempted, she will be far more receptive than otherwise. It is well to learn, right from the beginning, that foreplay is essential for the female (and usually this means manual stimulation of the area surrounding her clitoris) if she is to enjoy satisfactory sex. So often a boy mistakenly thinks, probably because the girl's vagina feels so pleasurable to him, that it also feels as pleasurable to her.

Actually, the vagina has very little sensation for her compared with the sensation she feels when her clitoral area is stimulated. A girl's clitoris is very much like a boy's penis. Without actual contact and friction in sexual activity, the girl is let down. If she has been sufficiently built-up before penetration and if the boy knows how to maintain contact with her clitoris after penetration, she stands a fair chance of participating in his sexual excitation and pleasure. Otherwise, she is likely to be left behind on the road to orgasm and is also likely to grow bitter about it after a while.

A boy and a girl must learn each other's responses, must know when and how to start the intercourse phase of their lovemaking without breaking the mounting excitation pattern of either partner This takes artistry. If a stimulatory pattern is interrupted the girl is likely to lose her momentum toward orgasm. One way to prevent this is for the boy to learn how to enter her near the beginning of their lovemaking from the man-above-woman-below position, then for the boy to shift slightly onto his side. In this position a boy can lie quietly inside while he plays with her clitoris with his hands. Thus he can feel her mounting tension as orgasm draws near and can begin his own in-and-out movements when he is sure that she has reached the point of no return. Thus they can move on into orgasm together.

However, they should not expect simultaneous orgasm in the beginning. Such an experience is the happy exception, not the rule, for neophytes. Lucky they are if each can come to orgasm, one at a time, in these early stages.

One gynaecologist tells her patients to "rock and roll" if they would maintain penile-clitoral contact. What she means is that all too often people don't know how to move their pelvises. They proceed with intercourse like two ironing boards banging together instead of like supple, mobile animal bodies that can reach toward each other with their pelvises.

The trick here is for a girl to practise this: Lie on a couch on your back with your legs apart, knees bent, and feet flat on the couch. Imagine a body six inches above yours and, keeping most of your back flat on the bed, lift the lower part to meet the imaginary body above it.

You may be stiff at first, but perseverance in this simple movement develops a skill which is important for good intercourse.

Another technique which should be learned is how to breathe. Most people breathe without experiencing any sexual feeling, yet breathing can augment the orgasm reflex. In any event, the full release of the breath is essential at the moment of orgasm, and the way one uses one's breath in lovemaking can make a vast difference to the total lovemaking experience. If you *exhale* fully with no muscular tightness interfering with the free flow of circulation from the centre of your body out to the periphery, you will feel warmth radiating into your hands and feet. For this to happen you will have to relax tension particularly in your groin as well as in your throat, chest, diaphragm, abdomen, buttocks, and anus. The muscles of reach are located in your groin and in the pectoral area, just where your arms join your body in front at the shoulders, and these will feel alive and pulsating if you are exhaling fully.

Here's how you can practise breathing:

Lie flat on your back on a soft bed and before you try any breathing techniques, do this: Kick your legs up and down hard and bang your arms against the bed. Bounce your head up and down on the pillow too if your neck feels stiff. If you feel like screaming, do so. You will look and act very much like a two-year-old child in a tantrum, but do it even though you feel silly, until you are out of breath and limp as a rag. This releases any tension relating to anger which you have unconsciously retained. It will also have you panting. Now sigh audibly, exhaling as fully as you can.

If someone sits facing you as you lie prone, with the palm of his hand in contact with your groin (fingers pointed up toward your heart), he will feel a sensation under his palm much like an air bubble passing under water, and your skin surface will feel warmer to his hand as you exhale. *You* will feel a streaming sensation, much like a gentle electrical current passing through the groin down your legs to your feet. The bottoms of your feet will begin to tingle, radiating warmth. The palms of your hands will also feel warm and glowing. Now this is fine. When you can create such sensations you are well on your way to the physiological condition which can lead to orgasm in your lovemaking.

The above phenomenon is difficult to describe. Nevertheless, if you practise patiently you will discover a delightful sensation which I have come to identify with a sense of sexual well-being. I became aware of it first during classes in natural childbirth where women were taught breathing techniques which lessened their perception of pain. Many of the women would report not only the reduction of discomfort, but the presence of a delicious form of sensuous pleasure which they could only describe as sexual.

Subsequently, I learned that full exhalation accompanied by full release of muscular tension can directly produce this sensation which is the usual prelude to orgasm. By breathing in this way a pleasant sense of well-being can be maintained for long periods of time in nonsexual contexts as well as sexual ones.

One further valuable technique to learn if you are a girl is how to relax and contract your vagina. To do this, imagine what you would do to keep from urinating if the comfort station were still ten miles down the road and you needed to use it. This is a fairly familiar physical experience and it is only a step from this to learning how to contract the vagina. In fact, the vagina automatically does contract when the urethra and the anus are tightened.

To make sure that the muscles of the vagina are working, you can insert your own finger into your vagina and contract around it. It will feel to your finger as if a glove were being removed. This little exercise is given to most women to do many times a day after they have given birth as it strengthens and tones the muscles of the vagina. It also tends to prevent the low back pain so common to many women. However, its chief advantage lies in its erotic implication, for it is not only sexually beneficial to a girl to have good control of her vaginal muscles, but it gives the boy with whom she is having intercourse a sensation that is thoroughly enjoyable to him.

People utter all kinds of sounds in their lovemaking, some quite frightening to the uninitiated. Your whole being tends to open up under intense sexual excitation and this includes the throat and the vocal chords. Whatever throat constrictions you have may burst forth as you release sexual tension. This may be a groan, or a sigh, or an exultant shout, but whatever it is, it is nothing to be afraid of.

In lovemaking it is important to verbalize your feelings and your desires to the beloved. This is often hard for beginners. A girl tends to feel that a boy should know everything she wants or needs without her giving voice to her wishes. This is nonsense, of course. A boy is apt to respond with, "Look, I'm no mind reader!" Thus lovers must learn to express themselves to each other. A boy especially appreciates this because he can then move more effectively to provide his beloved with that which will *really* please her.

Women tell me that what they value most are verbalizations of approval, of love and appreciation from the beloved. American men are not very skilful at this, but it is an excellent habit to develop early and to continue developing throughout life. A boy and a girl might start by sharing love passages in literature. Read these aloud to each other so that the words don't sound so unfamiliar or even downright foolish in your mouth. I've talked to men who have said they couldn't even form the words of love because these "sound silly". Yet they are the very words that excite and involve the woman in her deepest pleasure-giving responses.

Another way used by American boys and girls to show their love is through kidding, often by saying the opposite of what they really mean, both partners being fully aware of the jest. Boys especially seem to find it easier to express tender feelings by a negative rather than a positive verbalization. Nevertheless the meaning is transparent.

In intercourse one partner often arrives at orgasm before the other. When this occurs it is important for the one who has "arrived" to go on aiding the other until she (or he) has also been satisfied. This is sometimes difficult for a boy who no longer feels like doing anything but curling up and relaxing in his beloved's arms. Yet he will discover that if there are many episodes in which he finds satisfaction and she has not, she will grow so disinterested in sex that she will begin to make all manner of excuses for not making love at all. The average boy takes two or three minutes to come to climax. The average girl, probably because of cultural conditioning, takes thirty minutes. This may give you an idea of how important adequate foreplay is for the girl.

An experienced lover learns how to bring the partner to climax even after he has come to orgasm himself. Usually he can do this with his hand if his penis has become too flaccid.

It is not difficult for a girl to go on after her primary orgasm for she may well have a second or third orgasm, enjoying the experience all the while. This is one of the good reasons for petting a girl right to climax at the start, for she will still be quite capable of receiving the boy's penis and bringing him to orgasm while enjoying a second one of her own.

A girl generally feels a sense of loss if a boy withdraws too soon after orgasm. These moments may be the most precious part of the experience for her. She feels fused into oneness with him. For her it may be the time of all times for quiet talk. On the other hand, many boys want to roll over and go to sleep about then, but to a girl this says, "He doesn't care about anything but his own pleasure. He doesn't care about me."

If he does feel so utterly sleepy that he must drop off, he might at least reach out and hold his partner in his arms rather than turning his back to her.

When young men and women are ready to have intercourse, they are also ready to study thoughtfully one or more of the many good sex manuals which are available (see Bibliography). These are replete with instructions for improving technique. But all the technique in the world will not substitute for the strong flow of love that must exist if sexual intercourse is to be at its best. The ever-renewing quality of that love is what gives sexuality its power to heal and to bless. Without it sex is ashes in your hand once the moment of physical climax has passed.

More than that, there is such a thing as the law of diminishing returns. This law states simply that when any stimulant is repeated frequently enough it ceases to have the same impact as it did in the beginning. Sexuality can and often does behave according to such a law. It grows dull unless it is a true expression of an ever-deepening ever-creative love. In the crucible of such love sexuality results in continuing rebirth and renewal, and is never dull.

CHAPTER 5

Birth control

TODAY the world has about three billion people to feed and half of them are going hungry. If the present birth rate is maintained the population of the globe will have doubled in forty years and is expected to reach the twelve billion mark within seventy-five years. Perhaps, through technology, this surging mass of humanity can be fed, clothed, and housed, but in the end there will still remain the problem of space to live, space for children to play, and space for adults to enjoy some recreation too.

Obviously, in today's world it is a privilege but not a duty to procreate. Only those who truly love children and are prepared to care for them have any business giving birth to them. Furthermore, you who have decided to consummate your love in intercourse must especially give thoughtful consideration to birth control, for on orderly preparedness depends much of the happiness and success of your union. This is not to say that deep love between man and woman cannot expand to receive a baby at any time, but planned-for babies have the best chance of being given those educational opportunities that will prepare them to deal with life.

The method of birth control that you choose must depend on your knowledge of your own psychological makeup as well as on the degree of your need for protection.

If you are one of those who prefer to be swept off your feet during the moments before an act of lovemaking; if, in other words, you want to cast thought to the breezes and cannot brook even a momentary interruption, or cannot tolerate the thought of self-protection at that time, you will be safer with one of the newer contraceptives such as the pill, or an intrauterine device. On the other hand, if you are sufficiently motivated *and* have learned the discipline of thinking *as* you act, you can use any number of methods with relative security.

Furthermore, just *having* a method of birth control handy is no guarantee that you will use it when needed. Too often, in a moment of passion, you convince yourselves that God and the angels will take care of you and that somehow you will be able to solve tomorrow's problems when they turn up. Unfortunately, when the next menstrual period fails to appear, panic sets in along with the grim realization that the two of you have taken on more than you are ready to handle.

I repeat, if you are the impulsive type, by all means choose a form of birth control which can be effected at a time far removed from the act of sex, when your brain can function reasonably without being influenced by your emotions.

In choosing a satisfactory method you may find that the two of you have personal idiosyncrasies which incline you to one form in preference to another. For example, *you*, the girl, may have no timidity about handling your own genitalia, while another girl who has been brought up with greater strictness may be terribly shy about this idea. *You* might choose a diaphragm because it gives you more immediate control of your own body; *she* might prefer to have her lover use a condom. Or you both might prefer the pill in any event.

Religion may enter the picture. Roman Catholics, for example, have been limited to the use of the rhythm method. Many Catholics today, however, are using the pill as well as other forms of birth control with the honest conviction that their church is moving toward realization of the necessity of limiting the world's population, in spite of the opposition of some of the hierarchy. Even after the Pope's recent encyclical, many priests are referring girls to birth control clinics when certain conditions exist. Catholic girls should know about these exceptions, which are as follows: Since the rhythm method depends for its effectiveness on predictably regular periods, a girl cannot use it if her periods are not predictable or regular. Therefore, *if* she uses the pill to regulate her periods, many priests will consider this as allowable. Also it may be prescribed for her if she suffers from gynaecologic disorders, such as painful menstruation or premenstrual tension. Here the sequential form of the pill (more about this later) is usually prescribed by a physician to alleviate these conditions. As an *added* bonus she achieves a perfect form of birth control, though this, according to Catholic teaching must not be her primary motive – or, indeed, her motive at all.

Other factors may determine the form of birth control you use, such as how absolute your protection must be, which for the unmarried is 100 per cent.

Dr Robert B. Greenblatt, in an article prepared for the World Book Encyclopedia Science Service, says that among married women in the United States who use no birth control method at all, 80 to 90 per cent will become pregnant within one year. He goes on to say that of those who use the rhythm method, 40 per cent will become pregnant; of those who use diaphragms or condoms, 15 per cent will conceive; of those who use intrauterine devices (including, of course, only those women who can tolerate them) only 2 per cent will become pregnant; and of those who use the pill, none will conceive.

It is worth mentioning here, however, that the effectiveness of all methods, especially the diaphragm, is greatly increased by intelligent and precise use. Diaphragms, for example, can be 90 per cent effective in the hands of girls highly motivated and trained to use them correctly.

Dr Greenblatt's conclusions are substantiated by all research studies. It is pretty clear evidence that *if* it is absolutely imperative that you have perfect protection, the pill is obviously your answer, but it should only be taken under a physician's supervision.

I might add at this time too that for those who must lock the barn door after the horse has been stolen, there is a method of birth control called the "morning-after" pill.

Use of the morning-after pill must be started within three days of the unprotected intercourse. This means that a girl must promptly go to a doctor who is willing to prescribe medication for her. There are several possible morning-after drugs – all estrogens. Each obstetrician will have his or her personal preference for which preparation to use and its dosage relative to your needs. The first dose he may prefer to give as an injection. The important thing is that you go to him the day after the event if possible, and no later than the third day after.

Now getting back to the use of the pill, it is estimated that several million American women are regular users of oral contraceptives and that usage grows daily.

The Food and Drug Administration officials, as well as most physicians, are agreed that on the whole they are safe for most young women to take under a doctor's guidance. Some recent studies, however, seem to indicate that the incidence of blood clotting is slightly higher in users of the pill than in nonusers. Also there is some evidence of emotional changes including depression.

Although a few women experience other unpleasant side effects when they start taking the medication, these generally disappear fairly quickly. When women who have been using the pill wish to become pregnant, they are able to do so readily after discontinuing it. Babies born to these women are normal at birth and continue to develop normally.

There are some advantages of the sequential form of the pill over the older forms of the pill.

(1) It seems to act in many instances as a therapeutic agent in the relief of premenstrual tension and of menstrual pain.

(2) There appear to be fewer instances of a vaginal infection known as monilia among users of the sequential pill than among users of older forms of the pill.

(3) There are fewer instances of skipped periods, and furthermore, very few patients on this regimen report either an unusually scanty flow or an unusually heavy flow. Over 95 per cent report that their flow is "just like normal".

(4) There is even some evidence to show that for the girl with acne, sequential therapy frequently performs wonders. In-

hibition of ovulation in these patients seems to diminish oiliness of the skin and the tendency to form acne eruptions.

Those of you who are Roman Catholic may be interested in what a Catholic doctor stated at the thirteenth annual meeting of the American College of Obstreticians and Gynaecologists held in San Francisco in April of 1965. Said Dr James Beaton:

I have had very good experience in regulating menstruation, using Oracon. . . . Many of my patients had previously been given a combination product. Even though this conflicted with their religious viewpoint, they took it for a while. Then finally, they came to me in desperation, wondering if there wasn't something that would be more natural. This reflects the wonderful feeling about something like 'sequential.' I like the word very much. When I explained to my patients that sequential regimen consisted of an estrogen, which is the hormone secreted in the first half of the menstrual cycle, followed by a combination of an estrogen and progestin to simulate the latter half of the menstrual cycle, they liked and accepted it. I think this is probably one of the reasons why I didn't have much trouble with nausea, break-through bleeding or psychological disturbances.

However, if you are a Catholic but have no gynaecologic reason for using the pill (irregular periods, painful menstruation, or premenstrual tension), you will want to know the latest developments in the use of the rhythm method, unreliable though it is.

The rhythm method, to be effective at all, requires the greatest personal discipline and motivation, as well as careful education, preferably under medical supervision.

Actually, the rhythm method is *timed abstinence*.

According to Dr Alan Guttmacher, in his manual *The Complete Book of Birth Control*, the principles underlying the rhythm method are as follows:

"The two and a half days during which a woman can become pregnant are the two days before ovulation and the half day after it. In order to utilize the rhythm method, therefore, it is necessary to figure out *exactly* when ovulation is going to take place."

Unfortunately, since there is no precise way yet to tell exactly when a woman will ovulate, she must rely on estimates which are little better than informed guesses. Furthermore, a woman's period will vary considerably depending on factors such as fatigue, sickness, anxiety, etc.

To make allowances for these variations it is necessary to lengthen the time of abstinence. Dr Guttmacher's recommendations are as follows:

(1) Keep a written record of menstrual cycles for twelve consecutive months. Count the first day of menstruation as day 1 of the cycle, and the day before the next period as the last day of the cycle. At the end of twelve months, figure out how many days were in your shortest and how many in your longest cycle.

(2) Subtract 18 from the number of days in your shortest cycle. This determines the first fertile, or unsafe, day of your cycle.

(3) Subtract 11 from the number of days in your longest cycle. This determines the last fertile day of your cycle, or the day on which your unsafe period ends.

Because this formula, as you can see, requires a very careful set of calculations which many girls will not undertake, there have been a number of devices put on the market to make this simpler. However, it must be remembered that these so-called simpler calculations are also less accurate. There is really no substitute for the year's menstrual record. Furthermore, as Dr Guttmacher so wisely adds, "From adolescence on a record can be very useful when later you want to become pregnant and at some point it may be important to your physician in medical evaluation."

Frankly, I think that the rhythm method has no place in the lives of those who are not prepared to welcome a child, for its effectiveness is far from 100 per cent.

Perhaps the contraceptive that has had the most attention in recent years is the *Intra-Uterine Device* – commonly called the IUD.

Its success offers great hope in the solution of the problem of world population – particularly for underdeveloped areas.

The idea of intrauterine devices as contraceptives has been around for some time. However, in the past the majority of gynaecologists had rejected them because of the number of negative effects with which the early devices were associated.

However, from two widely separated countries, Japan and Israel, reports began to drift in of successful use of modifications of the earlier devices, and those modifications have been further developed and sufficiently tested in the United States so that IUD's have been released for general use.

The IUD's are objects made of plastic in various forms. The best have appendages extending through the cervical canal into the vagina for easy checking and removal. They are inserted by a physician.

For women who are able to retain them, the intrauterine device is highly effective. Its advantage is that it can be left in place indefinitely and not removed until pregnancy is desired or until the advent of menopause.

There are a few difficulties with them, however. Spontaneous expulsion has occurred in about 10 per cent of the women participating in the research studies. This spontaneous ejection ordinarily occurs during the first or second menstrual period after insertion. The use of an IUD with a tab or "tail" is important, so that a woman can check frequently on whether the device is still in place.

Another difficulty is that some women experience side effects, such as cramps, bleeding, or other discomfort. Ten per cent of the women participating in the research studies have reported such effects and have had to have the device removed.

But for the estimated 80 per cent who *are* able to retain them, the intrauterine device may prove to be closer to ideal than any other contraceptive because of its low cost, high effectiveness, and simplicity of insertion. (Always by a doctor, however.)

The unmarried girl however, will find that most physicians will not fit her for an IUD, at least not until after the birth of her first baby.

In any discussion of birth control we must not neglect the older so-called traditional methods which have been and are still reliable.

The *vaginal diaphragm* must be fitted by a doctor. If used by itself it does not guarantee complete protection, for, however carefully the type and size of cap are chosen for you by your doctor it cannot always prevent individual sperms from swimming past the circular rim of the cap. Because the vagina has soft, flexible walls, no cap can make a perfect fit. For complete safety, the diaphragm method of contraception *must* be a double one and an adequate amount of contraceptive cream or jelly must *always* be placed on *both* sides of the diaphragm. In this way the spermicidal cream or jelly catches sperm which escape the cream or jelly below the cap and swim past the rim into the upper part of the vagina. Theoretically, therefore, this method of contraception is safe and reliable, but faithful perseverance is needed and correct and careful use are all-important for although there are few diaphragm failures, there are very many human ones.

The best way to minimize the mechanical aspect of the method is to regard the few minutes necessary for the insertion and subsequent cleaning of the cap as one of the essentials of daily life, no more troublesome or time-consuming than brushing your teeth or combing your hair. If you insert the cap some time before every occasion when you are likely to have intercourse, then it will not seem like an unwelcome interruption and it will soon become a regular and automatic habit separated in time from the act of lovemaking. The cap should be inserted well before intercourse as a matter of convenience and *must not be removed until at least eight hours afterwards as a matter of safety.*

Compared with the cap-and-spermicide method, the various brands of *vaginal foam* on the market provide somewhat less safety. Each kind of foam contains a sperm-killing chemical, while the foam itself is designed to entangle the sperms and so prevent them from entering the womb. The absence of a mechanical barrier however, obviously diminishes the safety of the method. All brands of foam can be bought from a chemist's without prescription. Some are packaged in aerosol bottles and foam up when inserted in the vagina. When it is to be used the top of the bottle is opened and the applicator is placed over the top. Slight pressure triggers the release valve and white aerated cream is forced into the syringe, pushing the plunger out. It has several advantages over creams and jellies that have been designed as spermicides. It is less expensive to use then these, and the leakage after use is less than after the use of nonaerated creams and jellies. Also it is more effective as a method of birth control than the jellies and creams.

The condom has been, and still is, a reliable contraceptive, though many couples reject it because they feel that it reduces sensation for both partners. However, properly used it is highly effective as a contraceptive and it has the added advantage of controlling the spread of infection from one sexual partner to another, as for example, when the girl has vaginitis, or the boy has a chronic infection in which a tiny parasite, the trichomonas, causes vaginitis in his partner. (These are not venereal diseases, in the sense of syphilis or gonorrhoea, but may be very irritating just the same, and their eradication may take many months. They are, of course, to be avoided if possible, and the condom thus may be particularly valuable here.)

To ensure maximum safety, the condom should be put on before any sexual contact, since sperms are often released before ejaculation. You should hold the teat, if it has one, between forefinger and thumb to expel air and then unroll carefully over the full length of the erect penis. Each condom should only be used once and you should withdraw soon after ejaculation, carefully holding the condom in position on the penis. For extra safety condoms may be used in conjunction with a spermicidal cream or jelly.

Some couples who wish never to have children may choose sterilization as a permanent form of birth control. Sterilization does not interfere with the pleasure of either partner in intercourse, but it makes the one on whom it has been performed permanently unable to produce a child.

In men the operation is done by means of a minor and harmless surgical procedure. A short section of the vas deferens – the tubes which carry the sperm from the testicles – is cut and the remaining ends tied. Thus no sperm are present in the semen when the man ejaculates. This operation is called a vasectomy.

In the woman sterilization is achieved by having the Fallopian tubes tied and cut in a surgical operation known as a tubal ligation.

This operation must be done in a hospital under full anaesthesia and is much more complicated than vasectomy is for a man. Therefore, if couples desire permanent sterilization it is usually much simpler for the man to undergo the operation than for the woman.

It is possible to undo both operations by a further procedure, though there is only a 50–50 chance of success. Most persons don't consider sterilization unless they are very sure that they do not want more children.

Emotional factors play a very large part in the effective use of any kind of birth control. Whether a given method works or does not work may depend on reasons which have nothing to do with the efficiency of the methods itself.

For example, "accidental" pregnancies occur when girls, in their deep-down, so-called "unconscious" selves, want to be pregnant even though they have verbally agreed to the practice of birth control.

Doctors Hans Lehfeldt and Henry Guze have conducted a study of the psychological failures in birth control and have coined the phrase "willful exposure to unwanted pregnancy" or WEUP for short. Apart from such factors as shyness, anxiety, and poor emotional conditioning, they observed that a number of "accidental" pregnancies occurred which were really planned in order to force marriage. Both male and female partners have resorted to this stratagem. There has also been deliberate deceit by the female, accomplished either by clandestine omission of the diaphragm or by the claim of female sterility.

Dr George Devereux writes in a report on psychologic factors in birth control: "Both men and women tend to feel that the one who uses contraceptives, openly admits the presence of strong sexual impulses, which in our society, takes courage and a certain capacity to ignore social conventions."

This is especially true of girls who grow up in a strict Puritan tradition. It is one of the reasons why so many girls strenuously insist that it is the man who must use contraception.

Dr Devereux goes on to point out that some individuals, both men and women, resist the acquisition of contraceptives because they are afraid of coitus and the human closeness that goes with it.

If you are one of these, by all means consult a marriage guidance counsellor so that you may have professional help in overcoming this handicap.

Dr Devereux also has found that all types of inadequate contraception may be motivated by unconscious and largely self-punitive or aggressive impulses, including going to a family doctor already known to the girl as being highly moralistic and negative about sex. Dr Devereux says, "The prime motivating factors in inadequate contraception are: masochistic brinkmanship, unconscious wishes to become pregnant, and aggressive impulses toward the partner."

His reference to masochism as it relates to the choice of a doctor is worth mentioning. As perhaps many of you have already discovered, not all doctors are adequately prepared or motivated to provide you with a reliable method of birth control. Some doctors, either for emotional or religious reasons, or because of lack of training, are not so equipped.

If you have difficulty in finding a doctor who is able and willing to give you the proper instruction and assistance, get in touch with the Family Planning Association, 27-35 Mortimer Street, London W.1. They will be able to advise you of the nearest clinic. Some clinics do accept the unmarried though not all. At least they can give you the names of doctors in your area who can help you if the clinic cannot. (In a later chapter there is a discussion of ways to get the most help from medical and other professionals.)

If you wish to talk over psychological aspects of various forms of birth control, or other problems related to sexual love, by all means arrange for a consultation with a marriage guidance counsellor. You can obtain the name of a reliable one by writing to the Marriage Guidance Council, 58 Queen Anne Street, London W.1.

Remember that the time to educate yourself about birth control is *before*, not *after* you have intercourse. Otherwise you may indeed be like the farmer who locked his barn door after his horse was stolen. Examine your own motivations with care, making sure that your selection of a method and your decision to use it coincides with your real desires. If what you desire and what your partner desires are at variance, this might be a good occasion to visit a marriage guidance counsellor who will help you to iron out your differences. This is far better than using some method underhandedly to obtain your wish without your partner's consent. For with the counsellor's skill you will be more apt to arrive at a decision satisfactory to you both. Many girls may feel that it is the boy's job to provide birth control, and likewise many boys may feel that it is the girl's job.

Actually, it is your *mutual* responsibility.

The girl who is so immature that she still has to be taken care of as a baby, or the boy who cannot concern himself with their joint problem, is not ready for intercourse at all.

Remember too that only as each one of you individually solves the problem of the creation of children who are welcome, wanted, and prepared for, will the world's problems of overpopulation be mitigated.

CHAPTER 6

What can you do if you're pregnant?

By now you have gathered that when responsibilities are met, love expressed sexually can lead a couple mighty close to heaven on earth. However, when sexuality is shared without regard for the well-being of both partners, it can lead to the serious casualty of an unwanted pregnancy. Let's take a good look at this and then see how it can be faced should you have blundered into it before you knew any better.

You usually suspect pregnancy when you miss the first menstrual period after having intercourse. Don't panic – at the same time, don't let time slip away. The first thing to do is to make certain as soon as possible whether you really are pregnant or not. So, see your doctor and ask him to do a pregnancy test. If for some reason you don't want to go to your own doctor (and remember that he will treat everything you tell him in strictest confidence) or if you haven't got a doctor of your own, there are other ways you can have the test done:

(1) Telephone your local Family Planning Clinic (local addresses in telephone book or from Citizens' Advice Bureau, Family Planning Association national organization address in Appendix C, page 148) and ask whether they can arrange a test, for which they will charge about £1.50.

(2) Go to a chemist (a qualified pharmacist) who will arrange a test through a commercial laboratory, which will probably cost £2 or £3.

(3) Write to one of the laboratories that do pregnancy tests.

You will find advertisements for them on posters or in the newspapers.

(4) Write to the National Council for the Unmarried Mother and Her Child (address in Appendix C, page 149) and one of their social workers will tell you the easiest way to get a test done.

The drawback to (2) and (3) is that if the test is positive (which means you are pregnant), you may have no one to turn to when you get the result; whereas if you go to a doctor or Family Planning Clinic or contact NCUMC, there will be someone there to help you get over the shock and plan what to do next.

A pregnancy test is quite simple. You don't have to be examined. Simply take with you in a small, clean jar or bottle a sample of *your first urine of the morning*. You will usually get the result quickly, probably in about twenty-four hours. Sometimes the result will be sent to you direct; sometimes, the laboratory will want to send the result to your doctor.

You cannot have a pregnancy test done until your period is two weeks late (or six weeks from the beginning of your last period).

If the result is positive, you will know that you are pregnant. If it is negative, that will probably mean that you are not going to have a baby, though the doctor or laboratory may ask you to come back for another test a week or two later if your period still hasn't started, in case the result was inaccurate.

WHAT HELP IS AVAILABLE?

If you are pregnant you will need to think about making plans for the future. You may feel very frightened, distressed and confused, but try to keep as calm as possible and remember that there are plenty of people ready to help you.

Your family
Let us talk about your relationship with your parents, for you are

WHAT CAN YOU DO IF YOU'RE PREGNANT? 55

certainly going to need them if you find yourself pregnant accidentally. Usually, parents are the last persons to whom you wish to break the news, because you fear the news will hurt them. How often a boy or girl has said "it will kill my mother and father to know". Yet parents are the first people you should tell. Eventually they may have to know and they rarely, if ever, suffer the dire consequences you predict. Parents are tougher than you think, so tell them at once. This is one of the hardest things you may ever have to do; but after the first tears and anger have passed, parents can usually be counted on. Of course, they may be very upset and angry at first, since your news will be a great shock. They will be worried about you and your future. They may wonder if your pregnancy was partly the fault of the way they brought you up. But, just as your parents will take care of you after a motor accident, even though you have been at fault in your driving, they will care for you after the accident of an unplanned pregnancy. Remember that the baby you are expecting will be their grandchild and most parents would rather suffer the shock and unhappiness of knowing the truth than think that their child has been going through a very frightening experience without telling them and without giving them a chance to help.

You will need your parents as you have never needed them before. You will need their protection, their financial help, their experience in approaching people whose assistance you may need, and above all you will need them to support you emotionally through a time that can be exceedingly trying. You must remember, however, that most parents themselves don't know what to do at first, for most of them have never imagined that they would have to help you solve this kind of problem.

Sometimes, like you, they want to rush off and cry on the shoulder of their best friend. I hope they won't. The best counsel they can get will be from a social worker or from their doctor, priest or minister, provided that he is up to date and knowledgeable about such problems.

Especially if you, the girl, are very young, the attitude of your parents is a matter of great importance. Most girls are naturally reluctant to involve their parents and cause them pain or social embarrassment. If you are nervous about approaching them, a sympathetic doctor or social worker may be able to help you break the news to your parents gently. In their distress and anxiety, many girls forget that their parents may be unexpectedly willing to discuss the future of a potential grandchild. If adoption is being considered, then it is essential for you to ask your parents if they are willing to share in the maintenance of the child, before you make the final decision. For a girl without the support of her own family, doctor or employers, the advice and friendship of a social worker can mean the difference between despair of the future and a smooth and happy pregnancy.

Social workers
Even if you have told your parents and they are prepared to stand by you, do go to see a social worker as soon as possible. She will tell you what services you are entitled to, help you make practical arrangements and give you emotional support. You will also be able to talk to her about your wishes and plans for your baby. Most girls find it very helpful to talk to someone apart from their family and friends, who can see things from their point of view and who isn't emotionally tied up with the situation. The social worker can sometimes be helpful, too, in discussing matters with your family or your boyfriend. Don't forget, he may also need considerable help.

Unfortunately, it is sometimes difficult to find the social worker who can help you best. If so, ask your doctor or inquire at the local ante-natal clinic, or at the local authority Social Services Department. The addresses will be in the telephone book or at the Town Hall. The help available will vary according to the area in which you live. There are special social workers working for denominational agencies who are very experienced in helping unmarried mothers. Church of England social workers' addresses are often written up in the church porch. If you are Roman Catholic or Jewish, you can make inquiries at your own community offices or place of worship.

Assuming you do not want to go to a religious agency (these

WHAT CAN YOU DO IF YOU'RE PREGNANT?

are staffed by professional social workers whose aim is to help you, not to lecture you), you may get help from a social worker in the local Social Services Department or from a social worker at the hospital where you are going to have your baby. If you are living at home, your local health visitor will be a great support and will put you in touch with a social worker if necessary.

The National Council for the Unmarried Mother and Her Child will gladly give you information about where to go for help. If for any reason you don't want to make inquiries locally, or find it difficult, write to the NCUMC, 255 Kentish Town Road, London, NW5 (telephone 01-267 1361). Their social workers will respect your confidence and will write to you in an ordinary envelope addressed by hand, so that other people in the house will think it is a letter from a friend. NCUMC doesn't have social workers up and down the country and unless your questions are very simple ones, it will not be satisfactory to discuss things by letter only, so they will suggest the most suitable social worker to see in your own area. Do make an appointment with the person NCUMC recommends. If for some reason you don't want to, write to NUCMC and explain. The social worker there will suggest someone else, or if absolutely necessary, will see you herself. NCUMC can also help you in a number of other ways, depending on what you ask and need.

WHAT ARE YOU GOING TO DO?

Whatever your plans, don't let time slip away. Medical care is necessary whatever you do and definite arrangements have to be made. There are several courses open to you:

(1) You and your lover can marry.
(2) You can keep the baby and bring it up yourself with or without your boy's help and without marrying.
(3) You can have the baby adopted.
(4) You can have an abortion.

Let's consider these solutions.

(1) You can marry
Young marriages have many disadvantages and special hazards.

(*a*) If you are still being educated or being trained for a job, your education or training may be interrupted or cease altogether.
(*b*) Personality changes that go on in the late teens and early twenties are very great, so a couple who meet at eighteen may find they have little in common at twenty-two.
(*c*) The burden of supporting and bringing up a child may be too great for you to assume without help from your parents or some other source.
(*d*) You may have to start married life without a home of your own.

Sometimes, however, marriage is the best solution, particularly if you love each other deeply and if you and your boyfriend can find some way to complete your education or training. It simply is not true that so-called "forced marriages" are automatically doomed to failure. Many successful marriages have been launched prematurely; but anything premature takes special nurturing to ensure its survival.

(2) You can have the baby and keep it
To keep the baby takes courage. In order to bring up a child by yourself, you need a fair measure of stamina and to sacrifice quite a lot of personal freedom. Nowadays many more unmarried mothers keep their babies, but it is not an easy decision. The younger you are the more problems and difficulties you may have to face, especially if you are economically dependent on your parents. Again, you may think adoption is the right solution at first, then change you mind later. Or you may feel capable of caring for a little baby, but have fears about managing an older child or adolescent. In any event, whatever your fears and problems, think things over very carefully for yourself. By all means discuss the matter with your boyfriend and family – but at the same time remember, whatever they advise, the ultimate

WHAT CAN YOU DO IF YOU'RE PREGNANT? 59

decision and responsibility are yours. A lot of people will want to give you advice. Nevertheless, it is for you to make up your own mind whether, taking your own personality and circumstances into account, keeping the baby or parting from him is the best answer both for him and for yourself.

If you want to keep your baby, remember that most unmarried girls who bring up their children marry within three or four years anyway, usually very happily. And if you both wish, you and your new husband can almost always jointly adopt your child.

(3) You can have the baby and give him up for adoption
This is a hard choice but sometimes the wisest, especially if you are very young and have not got your family behind you. The act of giving up a baby for adoption is one which takes great unselfishness and courage. However much a girl may realize that she is not in a position to provide a good home for her baby, however eager she is to get on with the life she was living before she became involved in an unwanted pregnancy, the personal loss to her when she gives her baby into the keeping of another always represents a degree of sacrifice, since the gift of life is as precious as any which one human being can make to another.

All too often we assume that unmarried mothers do not want their babies. This is rarely the case. A baby which becomes available for adoption is usually very much wanted by his natural mother although he has come into being without the sanction of society. The mother puts herself aside in concern for the baby's well-being. She believes that he needs a home in a social unit accepted by society, a home warmed by love, and so she gives him these gifts rather than claim her own pleasure in motherhood.

You should never make a decision about a child's future simply to get out of your immediate difficulties. It is much more important for him than that. If you decide on adoption it should be because you think that is the best solution for him. So do not be stampeded into making up your mind prematurely. It is not essential to get in touch with an adoption agency before the baby is born unless you want to do so.

Who can arrange an adoption? At present there are three ways in which a child can be placed for adoption. Discussion is going on, however, at the moment about adoption law and Parliament may make changes some time in the future.

(1) You can place your baby through an adoption society or through you local authority Social Service Department.

(2) You may place him through a private individual (known in law as a "third party").

(3) You may place the baby yourself with a couple whom you want to be his adopters.

It is, at present, possible for a member of your family to adopt the baby. If you later marry a man who is not the baby's father, you and your husband can adopt the baby jointly.

Adoption arrangements are free except that if you can afford it, you may be asked to pay for medical examinations for yourself and the baby. Adoption can be a very happy solution for your baby, but even though many couples want to adopt, they are not all necessarily suitable adopters. As a result the vast majority of adoptions are now arranged by adoption agencies or local authorities, since they have experience about choosing the best adopters for a particular child, and fewer and fewer parents arrange adoptions privately or place the baby themselves. There is also the advantage that adoption agencies appoint an individual case-worker to guide you through all the stages. That is why your social worker will probably encourage you to use an adoption agency or local authority rather than to arrange "third party" adoption privately. Third-party adoptions are, however, every bit as valid and many are very successful.

If you decide to place your baby through an individual citizen acting as "third party", do tell him or her to find out from the local authority Social Services Department what his respons-

WHAT CAN YOU DO IF YOU'RE PREGNANT? 61

ibilities and duties are and what medical certificates must be supplied.

Equally, if you decide to place your baby yourself with adopters, then ask them to get in touch with the local Social Services Department and the local Magistrates' Court or County Court so that they will know what to do.

Timing. A baby may be placed with adoptive parents any time after he or she is born, but it is vital for the baby, the adopters and yourself that before he goes to his adoptive parents you are absolutely certain that you want to part with him. It can be tragic for everyone if you change your mind and tragic for you if you make a mistake. It is, of course, important for the baby that he goes to his new parents as soon as possible, but it is equally important that you should have enough time to be certain of your decision. If you have any doubts (and doubts from time to time are quite natural) do confide in your social worker or the social worker of the adoption agency. They will advise you when and how you should part from the baby. There are a variety of possibilities:

(1) The baby stays with you until he is placed with the adopters.

(2) The baby goes to foster parents (or sometimes to a residential nursery) for a few weeks after you have left hospital.

(3) The baby goes to the adopters as soon as you leave hospital.

Which is the best arrangement? That depends largely on yourself. On the one hand, if you have no doubts, you may wish the baby to go straight to the adopters from hospital. On the other hand, you may want him to go to foster parents for a few weeks until you can be quite certain that adoption is what you want. Or you may prefer to keep him until he goes to the adopters, so you know that he has gone straight from your care to theirs. *There is no law about the age at which babies must be placed with adoptive parents.* Nevertheless, you may run up against one practical difficulty. Adoption agencies sometimes do not place the baby with his adoptive parents until he is about six weeks old. This is partly to give you time to be sure that adoption is what you really want and partly so that the baby can have a medical examination before he goes to his new parents (at present he has to have a blood test when he is six weeks old). If, however, you are absolutely sure that you want him adopted, he may well be able to go to the adopters much sooner.

Obtaining an adoption order. The next three months are the most difficult ones. The adoptive parents have to remember that the natural mother has the right to change her mind, and that an adoption order cannot be made until the end of that time. For, no matter when the baby goes to his adoptive parents, they must have him with them for a three-month probationary period before they can go to court and ask for an adoption order. Any time that they have the baby before he is six weeks old does not count towards this period.

You will, of course, have to give your consent before the adoption order can be made final. This means that you give up all parental rights over the baby in return for the fact that the adopters become responsible for him, just as if they were his natural parents. Adoption is quite different from fostering, where you keep your parental rights.

The procedure for you is slightly complicated at the moment (it may be changed some day in the future).* The adoption society or Social Services Department will look after the practical details, so you have no need to worry about them. Basically the procedure is as follows:

(1) The adoption agency will want you to sign a preliminary consent asking them to arrange for your baby to be adopted. The social worker at the agency will give you a note explaining exactly what the procedure is and ask you to sign that you have read and understood it.

*Procedures for adoption are different in Scotland. So if you are living in Scotland, you should ask your social worker about them.

WHAT CAN YOU DO IF YOU'RE PREGNANT? 63

(2) You will receive a form from the adoption agency which you will have to sign in front of a Justice of the Peace, or the clerk of a magistrates' or a county court giving your legal consent to adoption. You cannot sign this form before your baby is six weeks old.

(3) The court will appoint an independent person (called the Guardian ad litem in England and the Curator ad litem in Scotland) whose duty it is to see that the baby's interests are being properly looked after and that all the necessary consents to the adoption have been given freely. The Guardian ad litem, who is usually a social worker, will need to see you some time before the court hearing. He will get in touch with you; and if it is not possible for you to see him at home, you should ask him (or her) to arrange for an interview at his office.

(4) You will receive a form telling you the date of the court hearing, asking you if you wish to oppose the adoption and if you wish to attend the court hearing. Usually you will want to say "No" to both these questions and to return the form as quickly as possible.

(5) Once the prospective adopters have asked the court for a hearing you cannot take your baby away from them without the consent of the judge or magistrate.

No matter whether you are using an adoption society, local authority Social Services Department or "third party", do keep in touch with them so that they can contact you when necessary and so the adoption is not unnecessarily delayed.

Incidently, if you think that you may want your baby to be fostered before he is placed with adopters, save up all you can of your maternity grant, if you are eligible for one, so that you can pay the foster fees. If you cannot afford these fees, talk the matter over with your social worker and you may find that either the Department of Health and Social Security or your local authority will help you.

Whether you are going to have your baby adopted or not, his birth must be registered. You may have to go to the office of the local Registrar of Births, Deaths and Marriages or the Registrar may come round the hospital ward. If you have decided on adoption, ask for a long birth certificate as this will be needed by the court.

Should I see my baby? Although many people think that a mother who is going to have her baby adopted will be better off having no contact with her baby at all, personally I completely disagree with this point of view. Having gone through the process with dozens of unmarried mothers, I cannot remember one who did not grieve when the time came to give up her baby for adoption, whether she had had contact with him or not. Like an artist who needs to see what he has created, a mother needs the satisfaction of seeing the life which has come into being through her body. Usually a young mother, even one who decides that she is giving up her baby, reaches out for some consciousness of the maternal experience. She expresses incredible pleasure over her child's beauty and in his unique perfections. This gathering up and savouring of the emotions of motherhood seems to serve as a release of feeling, as a brief excursion into fulfilled maternity. Again and again, when it is over, I have heard a girl express her gratitude for the opportunity to enjoy, however briefly, the marvel of her own creation. She seems to be saying that it helps to exerience maternity positively and to appreciate the joy of motherhood, at least for a moment.

Nevertheless, this is a highly personal question, and one which you must decide for yourself; so if you feel you would rather part with the baby without seeing it, you should do so without any feeling of guilt or regret.

If you do think this is the best course, you may fear that the hospital will make you see your baby and look after him, even though you are going to give him up for adoption. Whether you are expected to do so will depend upon the hospital rules. Some hospitals allow a mother to choose whether she wants to see her baby or not; others unfortunately give no choice except in very exceptional circumstances. So, it is wise to find out the practice of your local hospital in advance, and if you are afraid that you may be forced to see the baby against your will, ask your social

WHAT CAN YOU DO IF YOU'RE PREGNANT? 65

worker or doctor to intercede with the hospital authorities on your behalf.

The baby's father. Often you, the boy, can and will help out. This does not mean that you ought to leave school or give up your training or further education, especially since in the long run you will be in a better position to support the baby if you continue your training or education. It does, however, mean that you can stand by your girlfriend and help her in every possible way during the pregnancy, even if you are not going to marry or you both want to break up the relationship, and you should try to contribute something towards the baby's support. Your financial responsibilities and your legal position are described in Chapter 7. You probably feel very guilty about what has happened and there is a temptation to run away from the situation and deny that the baby is yours. Nevertheless, most men today resist this temptation and recognize that creating a child is a very serious matter and at least as much the man's responsibility as the girl's. There may be all sorts of ways in which you can give your girlfriend the help she needs and later perhaps you may be able to take on some of a father's responsibilities. Many girls would rather keep silent and bear their burden alone than go through the humiliation of insisting on your help. However, you should share the responsibility so far as you are able to and you should realize that it is your job to give your girlfriend all the assistance you can, since both she and her baby will need it badly.

You may possibly find that your girlfriend reacts against you during pregnancy, and even though you want to help, she won't have anything to do with you. She may behave like this because she feels guilty about the pregnancy and feels the emotional need to blame someone else. So be patient and, provided you were genuinely fond of each other before the baby was conceived, you may well find she will accept you once again after the baby is born.

If your girlfriend plans to have the baby adopted and she is not married, she is the only person in law who has to give her consent. You can ask to be allowed to make your views known to the court and the court will take them into account especially if you have shown a real interest in your baby and have helped his mother financially. Also, the adoption society, Social Services Department or "third party" will probably want to see you and make sure that you are happy about the arrangements.

You can in law apply to the court for custody of the child, but custody is only given to the father on rare occasions when the court considers that he can make proper arrangements for the child's care and that it is in the child's best interests. Of course, if the baby's mother does not want to bring up the child herself and has no feelings of bitterness towards you, she may well offer no opposition if you apply for custody. But that is a fairly uncommon situation. You can apply to the court for access to your child, but remember that in deciding whether or not to grant you access the court must consider the child's interests as paramount.

(4) You can seek an abortion

Often on first learning of an accidental pregnancy a couple panic and rush off to seek information as to how an abortion can be obtained. Illegal abortion is one of the worst answers to a tough situation, though legal abortion may be the best. Let's consider the whole question of abortion.

The word has commonly come to mean the interruption of a pregnancy by artificial means. There is such a thing, of course, as spontaneous abortion due to natural causes. In fact, approximately ten to fifteen per cent of all first pregnancies end in spontaneous abortion.

An abortion performed by a doctor for the benefit of the mother is called a therapeutic interruption or therapeutic abortion. Throughout the world there is a great deal of controversy about legal grounds for abortion and the present legal situation differs widely from country to country. In England we have the Abortion Act of 1967. It gives four sets of circumstances, any one of which allows a surgeon to terminate a pregnancy. Put into ordinary language, the four legal grounds for termination of pregnancy are:

(1) That if the pregnancy is allowed to continue *the risk to your life* will be greater than if the pregnancy were terminated.

(2) That if the pregnancy is allowed to continue *the risk of injury to your mental or physical health* would be greater than if the pregnancy were terminated.

(3) That if the pregnancy is continued *the risk of injury to the physical or mental health of your existing children* would be greater than if the pregnancy were terminated.

(4) That there is a substantial *risk of the baby being born with such physical or mental abnormalities* as to be seriously handicapped.

Under our law you cannot have an abortion just because you want one or think that it is the best solution to your problems. The final decision is a medical one. Except in an emergency, two doctors, each of whom has examined you independently, have to recommend the operation and each of them has to complete a form clearly stating the ground or grounds on which they recommend termination. If you are under sixteen, you will normally also need your parents' written consent.

Abortion is not a matter to be undertaken lightly. Even if a doctor is willing to perform the operation, do think the matter over extremely carefully and decide what your real feelings are, since you will have to live with the decision and it can be a very agonizing one to make. If you have religious or deep personal views that make abortion unacceptable (as quite a number of people do) or if you want an abortion but are unable to have one, remember that there are other ways of coping with the situation and that, if after having had your baby you do not want to bring him up, he can still be adopted.

In fact, before you decide to have a therapeutic abortion you should, I believe, be able to answer the following questions with an unequivocal "Yes":

(1) Would having the baby so affect my future life that I would be seriously and permanently handicapped by the experience?

(2) Might the baby's life be jeopardized by the possibility of a serious physical or emotional handicap?

(3) If this were to be my only chance to have a baby, would I still want to go ahead with the procedure?

The decision for abortion must be reached promptly, preferably in the first month. No doctor wants to perform an abortion after the third month of pregnancy and most prefer to do so in the first or second month.

If, having thought things over carefully you decide to seek a termination, go and see your National Health Service doctor. If he considers that you have legal grounds, he will give you a letter of introduction to a gynaecologist at a hospital. He will usually telephone the hospital to make an appointment for you. Unfortunately, the facilities for a legal abortion under the National Health Service vary greatly from one part of the country to another. Also, there is sometimes an overwhelming demand for hospital beds and in certain areas hospitals can only give appointments to patients who live in their "catchment area". As a result, your doctor may suggest that the termination should be done privately at a registered clinic, which will probably cost between £60 and £150. If this is the case, no matter how desperate you are, don't be tempted to go to a "back street abortionist". An abortion performed without proper skill and care or without benefit of hospital conditions might endanger your life or health and make it impossible for you to have another baby. If you cannot have an abortion under the National Health Service, scrape together or borrow enough money to pay for proper treatment in a registered clinic.

Some doctors do not approve of abortion. If your doctor takes this view, ask him to refer you to someone else and, if he is unwilling to do so, seek the advice of your local Family Planning Association. There are also a few special organizations that you can get in touch with. In London, for example, there is a centre (The Pregnancy Advisory Service, 40 Margaret Street, London W1N 7FB, telephone 01-629 9575/6) where you can see a doctor and a social worker. It is open five days a week, but appointments should be made in advance because it is extremely busy. If possible, take a letter from a doctor; but if this is not practical, you can be seen without one. The doctors running the service have established relationships with gynaecologists all over London who are willing to accept cases that they recommend. Fees are kept low and compatible with the patient's financial situation. Or they can refer you to a nursing home where charges are very reasonable.

There is also a Birmingham Pregnancy Advisory Service (109 Gough Road, Edgbaston, Birmingham 15, telephone 021-440 2570). If a termination is not possible under the National Health Service, the Birmingham clinic will refer you to a nursing home with very reasonable charges.

When you visit the hospital or in the case of a private termination the doctor who has arranged to see you, make an appointment in advance and take your letter of introduction, if you have one, with you; also, do be ready to give the doctor *all* the details you can in order to help him make up his mind about your case. At a hospital the doctor will probably ask a social worker to see you so that she can prepare a report about your circumstances and he may refer you to the psychiatric department of the hospital too, since three of the grounds for abortion involve "mental health". If you are seeing a doctor privately he may send you for a second opinion and, if the second doctor agrees, will book you a bed at a registered nursing home.

Surgeons are now so skilled in performing abortions that the operation is quick and simple and does not necessarily mean more than twenty-four or forty-eight hours in a nursing home or hospital. However, you may need to stay longer in order to rest and get back your strength. So you should be prepared to do so if necessary and don't forget it takes a little time to get back to normal after any operation.

You will probably feel very relieved after you have had your termination. If you feel depressed or unwell, then or later, do go and see your doctor or seek help from a Youth Advisory Clinic or Brook Centre if there is one in your area (addresses on page 148-9) or from NCUMC, since you may need medical help or simply to talk things over with an experienced doctor or social worker.

What happens next? It can not be said too emphatically that you should get proper instruction about contraception straight away, whether you intend to continue the relationship which caused your pregnancy or not.

CHAPTER 7

If you decide to go through a pregnancy unmarried

DURING PREGNANCY

How will you feel?
DURING pregnancy some of you will experience profound emotional changes. So will the boy who made you pregnant. The fact that both partners do experience personality changes during this period is one good argument, of course, for postponing pregnancy even within marriage until each partner is well acquainted with the other's usual behaviour. Otherwise it can be very hard for the boy to know which personality he is dealing with in his girl, the one influenced by changes in hormonal balance due to pregnancy or the one which represents her during her normal non-pregnant state. It is equally difficult for the girl to know what kind of response is usual from her lover and what is induced by his anxiety about her pregnancy. Of course, at this stage all that both of you can do is recognize that pregnancy does bring changes in personality and make up your minds to be especially forgiving and understanding towards each other.

Each of you is likely to be anxious about many things related to pregnancy, and you may be downright afraid of a few. For one thing the boy may wonder if he really is the father of the baby even while hating himself for the thought. If he is still in love, he may also fear playing second fiddle once the baby is born. He may ask himself, "Will my girl still be my girl, or will her interests be swallowed up in the child and in her new responsibilities, over which I have no control?" It is not without reason that a boy worries about this, for sociological studies have shown that the birth of a baby is not only the first real crisis in the lives of most married couples, let alone unmarried ones, but that many relationships break up because they cannot weather the strain. It takes a high level of maturity in both a boy and a girl to be able to forget self enough to focus on the needs of a new individual. Sometimes one or the other still feels so hopelessly helpless that he or she cannot stand the idea of sharing attention with a creature even more dependent. Furthermore, many boys are understandably worried about being able to help support a fully dependent creature. Up till now, you, the boy, could always tell yourself, with reason, that your girl was potentially just as adequate a breadwinner as were you. Now you know the full loneliness of being economically responsible, at least in part, for your share in this misadventure.

You, the girl, on the other hand, are discovering that the emotional support your boyfriend gives you is the most important single factor affecting the serenity and the happiness of your life, even if marriage is not feasible. You look to him for emotional sustenance as you never have looked to anyone before, subtly demanding more of him in every way.

Your dependence is not entirely unjustifiable, for research indicates that the influence of a man's positive participation in his wife's pregnancy does indeed seem to influence nearly every aspect of her feelings about her new experience, and that women who enjoy encouragement from their husbands actually are freer from fear, freer from nausea, freer from persistent food cravings, and are more likely to be better mothers in every way. Why then wouldn't you, even more than married women, feel this dependence?

In the light of these and other benefits, a boy at this point might well ask, "What does a girl consider 'emotional support'? How can I treat my girl, even though I am not going to marry her, so that she will feel sustained and not let down?" This is a good question to ask.

Above everything else a girl wants the father of her baby to be pleased, even if they are not able to marry, when she tells him that conception has occurred. (Irrational as it may be, she still wants to know that some irrational part of him also rejoices in this miracle, even though it may be a social catastrophe for them both.) His genuine delight over the idea of her pregnancy is something she remembers forever. Even if (quite understandably) he feels anxious about how they will manage, she needs his assurance that they will cope. She also wants to be made aware of his tenderness and concern for her well-being. As the pregnancy progresses every girl wants her lover to show pleasure in the way she looks, at least privately.

Married girls who have wanted to be pregnant nearly always take a lot of pride in their changing shapes, many advertising their condition by wearing maternity dresses weeks ahead of any real expansion in waistline. An unmarried girl cannot always do this; yet she is not immune from the same exhibitionistic feelings of pride. Often her boyfriend is one of a very select few to whom she can show herself, so she is especially gladdened by his appreciation of the beauty of pregnancy.

It also gives a girl intense pleasure to have him share her joy in the movements of the baby. Many a pregnant wife has told me of the emotional warmth she experienced when her husband wanted to lie snuggled close to her at night so that he could identify with her more intimately as she experienced intrauterine activity. An unmarried girl longs for this also. So if the two of you can have some times when you simply snuggle in each others arms, it will prove a great comfort.

Some girls feel that they are intellectually sluggish during pregnancy. As one young college student described it, "The bovine reaction has set in. My world has closed in in direct proportion to my abdomen going out. At first I was concerned that becoming a mother had robbed me of all mental stamina, but later I didn't care, not even when an old professor told me to have my head examined because he found me doing needlepoint embroidery on a bath mat, after teaching me comparative anatomy and physiology."

This is the moment for you, the boy, to rescue your girl's flagging self-esteem with reassurances and diversion. One perceptive young graduate student wrote in a letter to his discouraged girl, who at the time was away in a home for unmarried mothers: "Darling, as you become more and more absorbed in this vastly important event that is taking place inside you, you must expect that you will have less need to run to every fire or to follow the latest blasts or counter-blasts of the politicians. I am sure that a few months after delivery you will regain your real intellectual interests. You will then be better able than ever to concentrate on whatever you consider of importance." Such insight and concern were of great comfort to this girl.

It is true that women are intensely interested in what is going on inside them; and a boy with the initiative to bring a girl a book on obstetrics or infant care will find his gift appreciated. Many married women speak nostalgically of the pleasure they felt when their husbands attended a course for expectant parents with them, or otherwise participated in plans for an educated parenthood. Believe it or not, unmarried couples have enjoyed this experience also.

If you, a sensitive boy aware of your girl's boredom, will hunt up external distractions for her such as light-hearted movies, or detective novels which intrigue her imagination from the very first paragraph, these will be very welcome gifts. You should never underestimate her intelligence, however, even when she proclaims that she is a dullard. You would be wrong indeed if you assumed that her awareness of people, or of emotional atmosphere, were anything less than acute.

Most pregnant women want the fathers of their children to be as physically close to them as possible during pregnancy. Even the most independent of females finds that she has a streak of dependence which emerges in her yearning for consistent and frequent contact with the man she loves. This is even more true for the girl who is carrying a child without the benefit of marriage. Above all she wants him to tell her that she is still sexually attractive to him (which indeed she usually is).

Intercourse during pregnancy
Actually, a girl's attitude about sex changes very little during

pregnancy, although some girls find that they have a lessened desire for intercourse and a heightened desire for "just cuddling". However, most loving girls want to be the ones to bring sexual fulfilment to their lovers, especially if the latter will accept noncoital forms of sexual expression. Obstetricians should not prohibit intercourse in pregnancy without telling a girl of the availability of other ways for sexual satisfaction and release from sexual tension. Such release is one of the very best things that could happen to any girl during pregnancy, as at any time. In unmarried pregnancy, if the girl is far from home and often far from her lover also, this can be very trying. Autoeroticism is certainly in order.

In my own experience with pregnant girls I have found very little change in basic sexual adjustment during pregnancy. Some may experience a slight decrease of sexual desire, and may feel rather bad if their boyfriends have to suffer sexual deprivation. Others may not mind at all, especially if their previous sex life was not very satisfactory. If a girl has felt a good deal of anxiety about sex before her pregnancy, she may tend to experience more nausea, more persistent food cravings, and more depressive moods and obsessive fears during this time than if she had previously established a satisfactory sexual adjustment. Furthermore, if she has had a happy sex life with her lover before pregnancy, she may find that she intensely wants him with her during labour and delivery, while if her sex life has been unhappy she may not want him around at all. Also the sexually satisfied girl is more likely to find pleasure in breast feeding and to do it successfully than the one who was unhappy in sex.

One very interesting finding which has emerged from the now famous research conducted by Dr William H. Masters and Virginia E. Johnson, authors of *Human Sexual Response*, is that pregnancy is not disturbed by sexual intercourse, not even right up to the moment labour begins. This finding is in direct contradiction to the edict that used to be handed out by obstetricians in the past, namely that there must be no sex during the last six weeks before, as well as for six weeks after delivery. Since one of the real problems between many couples during pregnancy is this sexual deprivation, Dr Masters' finding, which cuts the time of abstinence in half, is a tremendous asset.

Incidentally, a position that makes intercourse comfortable in spite of the woman's protuberant abdomen, is as follows: Let the woman lie on a bed with her legs extending beyond its edge and her feet supported by a chair or stool. Let the man kneel or stand between her outstretched legs. Alternatively she may sit on his lap facing him and straddling his legs. In either position she is in control of the depth of penetration and there is no pressure upon her abdomen.

Obviously, if you (the girl) care about your lover and want to continue your relationship with him, even if you do not intend to marry, you would be wise to enter into any kind of noncoital sex that pleases you both whenever you yourself are prohibited from intercourse. Not that a thoughtful boy would be unwilling to deprive himself, but deprivation tends to provoke unnecessary frustration and resentment. Resentment leaves the way wide open for tempting him into other relationships at a time when it may be most hurtful to have him desert you. The period right after birth will be a time of tremendous stress and strain for both of you, and it is also a time when sex must be prohibited to women. Furthermore, nature has so arranged a girl's hormonal balance that physiologically she is like a castrate for a while. It helps if a boy knows that his girl may feel and act disinterestedly at this time and that her disinterest is primarily due to lack of female hormones, and not to lack of love.

Anxiety and pregnancy
The evil witch of pregnancy is fear, whose ghost haunts the happiness of nearly every parturient female. Fear has even been held responsible for some obstetrical problems in delivery.

The most usual fears of pregnant girls are the following: fear of the birth process itself; fear of the unknown; fear of the baby's dying; worry about managing social, economic, or study obligations; sexual problems and worry about the boy and whether they will have a continuing relationship. If you, the girl, want to achieve a relaxed labour you must get rid of your fears of failure and inadequacy, and you must put away any negative superstitions that you may have acquired.

Perhaps something needs to be said about old wives' tales. You are not as burdened today as was your grandmother by fear-provoking stories, but there is plenty of evidence to suggest that prospective mothers are far from free of their influence. Curiously, very few of you will be told such tales by men. It seems to be one of the more unpleasant characteristics of the female of the species that she passes along such spine-chillers to other females. Childbirth education makes a fine forum for the airing of all kinds of beliefs, most of which turn out to be nonsense which you can then laugh at and discard.

A few of you may worry that a previous tendency to neurosis may break forth into a full-fledged psychosis during pregnancy or childbirth. Actually, the bulk of studies done on this subject indicate that, while childbirth may be a precipitating factor in a pre-existing dormant psychosis, it is highly improbable that childbirth will cause a real mental illness in those who have been merely neurotic. So if you feel unusually blue or if you sometimes want to "jump out of your skin" (as some girls have described their sensations), don't panic. Just ask for a good chat with your obstetrician and if he can't spare the time for emotional problems, go to see the sister or the social worker at the hospital.

Some girls experience excessive fear that has an obsessive character about it. Usually this is related to other experiences that have happened to them long before the pregnancy, usually in early childhood, and these have left a residue of guilt. For example, if you as a three-year-old girl wished your baby brother dead when he was particularly annoying (as most children do at one time or another), and then at a later time he actually did die, you may have felt that somehow you caused the death, and your unconscious may be burdened with guilt and fear that fate now will punish you through your own child. Sometimes an obsessive fear relates to excessive guilt over childhood masturbation because an ignorant adult converted the innocent act into a deadly sin.

Unidentified anxiety, when present, is often related to sexual frigidity. This is just one more reason for solving your sexual problems. Interestingly enough, normal healthy girls rarely fear death in childbirth, though a good many do fear the possibility of pain.

This might be as good a time as any to talk about the control of pain during delivery. Actually, with the help of modern medicine and childbirth education, very few girls need to experience anything more uncomfortable than a hard menstrual cramp. Some don't experience that much discomfort. Discuss any fears that you may have with the social worker at the hospital, the health visitor or a doctor or midwife at your hospital or local ante-natal clinic.

In courses that prepare you for childbirth you are taught how to breathe, how to relax one set of muscles while another set is working hard, and how to utilize contractions to the best advantage. In the absence of specific obstetrical complications, pain in childbirth usually comes about when:

(1) there is fear, creating tension which in turn results in pain;
(2) two muscle groups oppose each other in such a way as to obstruct the easy passage of the baby through the birth canal.

You will find it beneficial to go to classes at the hospital or antenatal clinic where you can learn about the physiology and psychology of pregnancy and how to do exercises to help control your breathing and muscles in order to make labour as relaxed and painless as possible. If there are no classes in your own area, you can contact the National Childbirth Trust, 41a Reeves Mews, London, W.1. (telephone 01-493 3605). This is their head office and London teaching centre, but they will also be able to give you names and addresses of centres in other parts of the country.

Childbirth education trains a prospective mother to minimize sources of pain and goes a long way towards eliminating fear. Many of the books which I have listed later in this chapter and in the bibliography help to explain the physiological and psychological side of pregnancy. Some hospitals and clinics show films or slides on childbirth.

Apart from the things you yourself can do to eliminate most of the discomfort from labour such as education and training, the doctor at the hospital is prepared to supply a variety of different analgesic and anaesthetic aids if needed. It is quite fair – indeed, I would suggest mandatory – to have a good straight talk with him about his practice in the matter of pain control. It is not enough for him to say to you, "Just let me worry about that, dear." More often than not such doctors have very unhappy patients at the time of labour. A conscientious doctor will tell you what methods he is most at home with, and what he is prepared to do. Furthermore, many doctors will go a long way in letting you have the baby in the way you want; in other words, will respect your desire for the degree of conscious co-operation that you are willing to give. But it is not fair to expect him to put you to sleep and have you wake up with a baby in your arms. Occasionally such a miracle does occur. Generally, however, some degree of co-operation is required of you, and it must be remembered that what knocks out the mother, knocks out the baby also, so there is a definite limit to the amount of analgesic relief that can be administered without harm to the baby.

The wise mother-to-be applies her time well during pregnancy to such training as will minimize the need for medication during childbirth, and then accepts with gratitude whatever modern medicine can offer in making childbirth easier and more pleasant.

Where will the baby be born?
It is important both for you and the baby that you should keep healthy and that you should receive the best care and advice from the earliest stage in your pregnancy. So get in touch with your doctor or your local ante-natal clinic *as soon as possible* and, as soon as you can, decide where the baby is to be born. If for some reason you need to change your doctor or don't have one, ask your neighbours or friends if they can recommend a good doctor or look up the list of local doctors at your nearest public library or post office.

Where can you have your confinement? There are several choices. If you have the money, you can of course ask your doctor to arrange for a private room in a hospital or in a clinic or nursing home. But few girls are in a position to do this. More probably you will want to go into a National Health Service hospital which has a maternity department.

One point will need considering – where will you live and work? In deciding where the baby is to be born you may be influenced by whether or not you wish to be near your family and friends.

If you decide to live away from your parents, perhaps you can stay with friends or relatives during the earlier months. There are also families who are willing to take in unmarried mothers either as paying guests or as home helps under the same sort of arrangement as foreign girls working as au pairs. Alternatively, a social worker in your own town will help you to find a home or hostel in a different part of the country. Once you have found a place to live, you may be able to hold a job until the last few weeks of pregnancy and to continue your college work or to learn a skill like typing which will help you to support yourself after the baby is born.

Mother and baby homes
Another possibility is to go to a mother and baby home.

Mother and baby homes in this country are not at present controlled by any central authority and information about them is not always easy to find. However, there is an excellent book by Jill Nicholson entitled *Mother and Baby Homes* and it is well worth reading before you decide to go to one. These homes care for unmarried mothers – including schoolgirls, teenagers and middle-aged women – during the later weeks of pregnancy and for a few weeks after the baby is born. There are about a hundred homes in Britain and they can be divided into two kinds, some being run by voluntary bodies (mostly religious and with a wide variety of denominations) and others by local authorities.

If you want to go to a mother and baby home, ask your social worker or NCUMC to help you arrange this. NCUMC has a directory of homes, but is it primarily designed to give social workers information about the homes, since a social worker usually makes the arrangements. Social work agencies in your home town should also be able to give you names of homes in different parts of the country.

You may find it very helpful to go to a mother and baby home, since you will have the comfort and company of other mothers and time to make up your mind without outside pressures about the really important question – do you want to bring up the baby or should you have him adopted? If you are planning to keep your baby, a stay of six weeks or so after he is born does have some advantages, especially if you are going back to a bedsitter or flat of your own, since you will have a chance to learn to feed and take care of him and to adjust to motherhood without the stress of having to fend for yourself.

Here perhaps I should give a word of warning. Mother and baby homes vary a great deal. Most are small and informally run, with nicely decorated rooms. A few are more like old-fashioned boarding schools with strict discipline and rather bleak buildings. The atmosphere depends mainly on the personality of the Matron. You should therefore find out all you can about the home you have in mind and it is best to visit it in advance, so you know what to expect and will be happy when you eventually go there.

In the past mother and baby homes expected a mother to stay for six weeks or until after the baby was placed for adoption. Most homes are more flexible nowadays and babies are often fostered prior to adoption or go straight to the adopters, but the Matron normally has the last say about admitting you. So, if you can't conform with her ruling, try to make other plans, even though no home or hospital has the legal power to make you stay longer than you wish. If you are worried, do discuss this with the social worker who is making arrangements for you, or with the Matron.

Before you go to the home, ask what your expenses will be. The local authority will normally subsidize or pay your fees, though this may be conditional on your contributing a substantial part of your maternity allowance. If you are not entitled to a maternity allowance and the local authority doesn't pay your fees either in full or in part, you may be able to get an allowance from the Supplementary Benefits Commission. However, normally they only pay about £4.50 towards the fees and £1.20 per week pocket money for yourself, plus a further £1.50 per week for the care of the baby if you return there after the birth. So, if the home charges more, you, your family or boyfriend will have to make up the rest. Many homes reduce the fees charged to a mother, if she can't afford to go there otherwise.

If you decide to go to a mother and baby home, contact a local social worker or NCUMC *before you leave your own home*. Otherwise, you may have difficulty in getting your local authority to pay the fees.

Continuing your education
If you are still at school or a student, don't assume that your education must be sacrificed. You will need the best qualifications you can get in order to find a good job, if you are going to bring up and support the baby yourself. If you are going to give him up for adoption, you will find it some consolation to have interesting and satisfying work. It is usually difficult to stay on at school if you are pregnant. Some schools will allow a girl to stay on if she can be discreet and do most of her work at home. Unfortunately that rarely happens, though your school may well be prepared to let you return after your confinement. Many girls, however, prefer to go back to another school or to a technical college or college of further education, if they are old enough.

Certain mother and baby homes cater specially for schoolgirls and provide full-time or part-time teachers. Others arrange for you to attend classes in the home or in the neighbourhood. So do discuss this with your social worker before you choose a mother and baby home. If you stay at home with your parents, you may be able to arrange for tuition through your local authority.

If you have left school and are at university or college, you will probably find most of the staff are sympathetic and are

IF YOU DECIDE TO GO THROUGH A PREGNANCY UNMARRIED 83

anxious for you not to give up your studies. However, the college may prefer you to leave until after your confinement and this may mean that your grant is suspended for all or part of the academic year, in which case you can get financial help from the Supplementary Benefits Commission as explained towards the end of this chapter. If exams are due during your pregnancy, your college may well allow you to stay on to take them, especially if they are your finals.

What about your confinement and medical care?
Your doctor will give you a letter of introduction to a hospital. The hospital will want you to attend for regular check-ups at first every month, then once a fortnight and eventually once a week during the later stages of your pregnancy. They will also give you advice about diet. Under the National Health Service you will receive exactly the same treatment as a married woman and your medical care and confinement will be free.

If you go to a mother and baby home, they will put you in touch with the hospital used by the home. Most homes arrange for confinements to take place at the nearest maternity hospital, although there are still a very few which also serve as maternity homes. Wherever you decide to have your baby, do attend your ante-natal appointments regularly.

There are some things you will want to find out about the hospital. For example, does it have "rooming-in"? This means that the newborn baby stays beside the mother's bed most of the time, instead of in a communal nursery. Many girls like this system, because they feel more at ease when they go home if they have seen what is happening to the baby all the time and have been able to participate in his care from the very beginning. If you plan to breast-feed, rooming-in has the great advantage that, having the baby beside you, you can feed him when he becomes hungry rather than when the clock says he should be. You are therefore able to adjust to one another's routine more easily and are saved from the anxiety of clock-watching, which can interfere with relaxed feeding. Other mothers prefer their babies to be cared for in the hospital nursery, feeling that their own much-needed rest will be interrupted by the demands of their new baby and the crying of other babies in the ward.

You will also want to find out if you are able to choose whether to breast-feed your baby or not; and if he is to be adopted, whether you will be expected to see and care for him. Hospitals vary in the amount of choice that they give to unmarried mothers. Some allow a mother to choose if she is placing her baby for adoption. Others will only agree that she should not see her baby in very special circumstances. Most hospitals encourage breast-feeding, but of course would not expect this of a mother who was parting from her baby.

It is becoming a common practice for husbands to be allowed to stay with their wives during labour. Many women find this a great comfort. Assuming this is the practice at your hospital, ask the sister beforehand and your boyfriend will be allowed to remain with you, if you wish. I might add that I have never known a father who, in witnessing the birth of his child, did not feel closer to both mother and child because of the experience and who did not find that participation in childbirth really is one of the most wonderful experiences in the world.

Maternity benefits

If you have been earning and have sufficient stamps on your National Insurance card, you will be entitled to maternity benefits. You can get the necessary application forms from your local Social Security office or from the Maternity or Child Welfare Clinic (your doctor, social worker or midwife will also have them). You will need a certificate of pregnancy to send with it and the doctor or midwife will give you one of these too. There are two maternity benefits – maternity grant and maternity allowance. At present the amount allowed is £25 for the maternity grant and £6 a week for the maternity allowance. You can claim the grant between nine weeks before you expect the baby and three months after he or she is born. The maternity allowance is normally paid for 18 weeks, beginning 11 weeks before the expected week of confinement, but not for any time when paid work is done. If you do not claim at the right time you may lose the benefits. Further details including when you should claim them are given in a leaflet 'Maternity Benefits' (NI 17A) obtainable from your local Social Security office. If you are very young and have not earned your living or have earned it for a very brief time, you will probably not be entitled to maternity benefits; but if you are not sure about this, do consult the local Social Security office. Your social worker will help you with addresses if necessary.

If you are working, ask your doctor how long you can continue, and stop when he advises you to. Pregnancy is quite a normal condition and if you feel healthy you will probably be able to go on working for several months. If you are entitled to a maternity allowance but have to give up work before it is due, ask your doctor to sign a sickness certificate and you will receive sickness benefit prior to your maternity allowance.

Supplementary benefit
If you are too young to qualify for a maternity allowance or find the allowance too small to live on by itself, you can get Supplementary Benefit providing your income brings you within its scale. You will be able to obtain an application form from your local Social Security office or Post Office. Unfortunately if you are not yet sixteen, you will only be entitled to Supplementary Benefit if your family is for some reason receiving it already. This may make life difficult for you, but there are ways of getting help and your social worker or NCUMC will gladly advise you. Some local authority Social Services Departments can give help too, but what help they are able to offer depends on the practice in the area in which you live.

Welfare foods and medicine
Pregnant women and nursing mothers are entitled to one pint of free milk a day if they have a low income. You can get an application form for a milk token book from your local ante-natal clinic, family doctor or health visitor. You then simply hand the milk token book to your milkman. If you are going to a mother and baby home, take it with you. Pregnant women and nursing

mothers whose income is low are also entitled to free vitamin tablets and orange juice, which can be obtained from your antenatal or infant welfare clinic or your doctor.* They too can give you a form in order to obtain free medicine, since all medicines prescribed by your doctor during pregnancy and the first year after your baby's birth are free of charge, and so is dental treatment. Consult the leaflet "Family Benefits – Your Right to Claim Them" or the local office of the Ministry of Social Security to find out if you are eligible.

Clothes and equipment for the baby
Before your confinement you will want to gather together equipment for the baby. Few things will automatically be given to you by friends, if you don't plan to tell them about your pregnancy till later, so get together the essential things yourself.

If you are going to bring up the baby yourself, you will of course need more than if he is to be adopted (if you are planning adoption, ask your social worker what you should get). You will want a cradle or cot for him to sleep in and a carrycot with wheels or a pram. If you can't afford a new one, your health visitor will probably know of cheap second-hand ones or you may be able to borrow one from relatives or friends. NCUMC sometimes have free second-hand ones. You will also need:

1 inexpensive baby bath;
1 or 2 pails with covers for dirty nappies;
1 plastic or rubber sheet for the cot and another for changing the baby on;
Several soft baby sheets and blankets;
3 dozen or so towelling nappies and some muslin ones;
Paper nappy liners;
3 nightgowns;
3 or 4 vests;
1 or 2 shawls (blankets can also serve as extra shawls and vice versa);

*All mothers can buy orange juice, cod liver oil or vitamin drops and vitamin tablets whether they have free tokens or not.

IF YOU DECIDE TO GO THROUGH A PREGNANCY UNMARRIED 87

3 babygrow suits;
1 or 2 warm coats (in winter);
2 cardigans or pullovers and trousers or pram suits (in winter);
Bonnet, bootees and mittens (in winter).

If you cannot afford the clothes you need, do ask either your own social worker, the maternity social worker at the hospital or NCUMC about this. You will also want to have on hand too such supplies as:

Sterile cotton wool balls and buds;
Safety pins;
Baby oil, cream, soap, powder and shampoo;
A jar of zinc and castor oil ointment;
1 or 2 feeding bottles and several teats (even if you do intend to breast-feed, since the baby will want water etc. Wide-necked bottles are probably most convenient for making up feeds and unbreakable ones have the advantage that later on the baby can safely hold them himself);
A bottle warmer (only if you can afford it);
Rose hip syrup;
Gripe water;
Hair brush and nail scissors (both are specially made for babies);
Possibly a rubber comforter or dummy;
Nappy sanitizing solution.

You may well need an airer or clothes horse (or perhaps a retractable clothes line that you can fix over your bath) to cope with drying all the baby's nappies and clothes. You will find that babies seem to need an endless stream of warm, dry, clean clothing! You must get a fireguard too, if you have any kind of fire.

Books on baby care
You should read some books on baby care. You may be familiar with Dr Spock's famous *Baby and Child Care*. One of the most interesting and informative books I have read and one which I

think you will find fascinating too is *Modern Motherhood: Pregnancy, Childbirth and the Newborn Baby* by Beth Day and Margaret Liley. Other useful books are *Your Wonderful Baby* by Willis J. Potts, *Preparing for Childbirth* by Frederick W. Goodrich and *New Childbirth* by Erna Wright. You will probably also find a leaflet called *For You and Your Baby* very useful, which is available from the Department of Health and Social Security or from your local authority Social Services Department.

BRINGING YOUR BABY HOME

Frequently a girl wonders how much help she will need at home after the birth of her baby. The answer is "All she can get". If you have spent your pre-natal months in a home for unmarried mothers, you may be able to return there for a few weeks until you get back on your feet again. Such homes often have staff who are very helpful and will teach you to take care of the baby. If you go home straight from hospital and are going to be alone, ask the sister or social worker if you can have a home help (you will probably have to pay for her according to your means). But in any event, find some way before you go in to hospital to arrange time to recuperate. For a month or more after your confinement do not even consider tackling a job and, if at all possible, do try to find a relative or friend to help you at least for a week or two.

You will need to conserve your strength for the care and enjoyment of your baby, as well as for your own future health. In a few months you will feel able to take on the demanding chores of your new world, but take it easy for those first few weeks if you can possibly arrange it.

Of all the privileges given to men and women, parenthood is one of the greatest. It stretches the body, mind and spirit and it rewards one in infinite excitement and satisfaction. If you are pregnant, even though you didn't plan it, you are in the process of launching yourself on one of the most meaningful experiences that life has to offer.

Like many new mothers you may feel a bit lost. If so, ring up your local health visitor; health visitors are trained experts on baby care. They can help with feeding problems or other difficulties that crop up as the baby grows older and will tell you when he should be immunized against various diseases. You can contact your health visitor through your local infant welfare clinic or the Public Health Department. Your doctor will have the address of the local health visitor too and may even have a health visitor specially attached to his surgery.

Financial support from the baby's father
You can take out a summons against the baby's father and apply to a magistrates' court for an affiliation order. You will have to give the court some proof that he is the father apart from your own word, such as letters from him or evidence from your friends or parents. Your social worker or the lawyer at the Citizens Advice Bureau will advise you, but do remember that you can apply for Legal Aid (which means the services of a solicitor, and if need be a barrister, either free or for a low fee). To obtain Legal Aid ask your social worker for the name of a solicitor, unless you happen to know a suitable one yourself, and he will tell you how to apply for a Legal Aid Certificate. If the case is proved, the court will decide how much the father should contribute towards your child's upkeep. Take out the summons *before the baby's first birthday*. Otherwise, unless the father was abroad at the time of the birth or has contributed voluntarily to your baby's upkeep during the first 12 months of his life, it will be too late. If you do not want to take your baby's father to court, provided that he is willing to pay maintenance, your social worker or a solicitor or NCUMC will advise you about making a private agreement. Your baby's father should consult his tax office about his liabilities before deciding how much maintenance he can commit himself to pay.

Accommodation
If you are to bring up the baby yourself, you will need somewhere to take him when you leave hospital. Even if you plan to live away from your family, you may find it helpful to go back to them for a few weeks while you regain your strength. Finding

accommodation may be your worst worry. If so, your local social worker will gladly help you and NCUMC can supply information about special flatlets for unsupported mothers. Unfortunately there are not enough of these to meet the demand, but it is well worth inquiring and you may be lucky enough to get one.

Most mothers go back to their parents' home. Even parents who refuse to have anything to do with their daughter before the baby is born, often change their mind when they see their grandchild and realize that their daughter really does intend to bring him up. Living at home will probably work out very happily indeed, but – especially if you return to work – you may have to make a firm arrangement with your mother about who does what for the baby. Otherwise both of you may feel resentful later, if she wants to take charge of him too much!

What other kinds of accommodation are there? Apart from the usual flats and furnished rooms to let via estate agents, newspaper adverts or cards in newsagents' windows, you can contact your local Housing Department and ask them to put your name on their list, although unfortunately there may be a long wait before you are accepted. Alternatively, there may be a family housing association in your area which accepts unsupported mothers or a branch of the Catholic Housing Aid Society (they house people irrespective of religion). If you live in the London area, you can contact Shelter, whose full address is Shelter Housing Aid Centre, 189a Old Brompton Road, London SW5, telephone 01-373 7276. If you find accommodation with a private landlord, then it is sensible to see that you have a rent book.

If you have difficulty finding a place to live, do ask your local Social Services Department or social worker for help and whatever happens try to keep your baby with you, as it is sometimes hard to get together again once you are separated.

What about money?

If you want to stay at home and look after your baby, you can apply for financial help from the Supplementary Benefits Commission, which is part of the Department of Health and Social Security. They are able to provide an allowance for you and the

IF YOU DECIDE TO GO THROUGH A PREGNANCY UNMARRIED 91

baby to live on and for your rent, provided your financial position brings you within their scale. They can also make additional payments for clothing, bedding and furniture in some cases. A leaflet explaining the scale of payment and other benefits to which you may be entitled can be obtained from your local Social Security office. It is called "Family Benefits – Your Right to Claim Them". If you are living away from home, you will be entitled to more than if you are staying with your parents. The amount increases when you reach 21; and you are entitled to draw Supplementary Benefit until your youngest child is 16, unless you marry or live with a man who is supporting you.

What happens if you go out to work? If you work part time, you can draw Supplementary Benefit; although, if you earn over £2 a week, your allowance will vary according to your earnings and your working expenses (including fares and day care for your baby). Full-time work disqualifies you from receiving Supplementary Benefit. There is a new allowance to which you may well be entitled if you are working full time and earn less than £18 a week. It is called "Family Income Supplement" and is certainly worth applying for, since in some cases it will be as much as £4 a week. For details inquire at the local office of the Department of Health and Social Security or from NCUMC.

Many mothers are faced with the dilemma of choosing between going out to work and staying at home to look after their children. You may perhaps prefer to work, both in order to make yourself more independent and so as to gain the stimulus of adult company and an interest outside your home. But, whatever you do, you must of course take into account what is best for the baby as well as for yourself. If you decide to work, you will need someone responsible to take care of your baby properly while you are away. If you are lucky, your mother may be willing to look after him for you or there may be a local authority day nursery in your area which gives priority to unsupported mothers and which will charge according to your means. Otherwise, your health visitor should be able to give you the names and charges of local day minders or private day nurseries.

Whether you are working or not, if you are in financial difficulties contact your social worker or NCUMC, as there are funds that can often be used to help mothers and children in need.

Registering the birth
All parents are now automatically given the new free short birth certificate, unless they specifically ask for a long one. The short birth certificate does not mention the parents' names and there will be nothing on it to show that you were unmarried when he was born. You will want to ask for a long birth certificate (which you will have to pay for) if the baby is to be adopted.

If the baby's father and yourself want the father's name entered in the birth register and his signature to appear on a long birth certificate, you will need to register the birth together. It may also be useful for you to know (for example if the father is unable to register the birth with you) that he can make the declaration in front of a lawyer, which with your consent enables the birth entry to be altered.

When you register the birth you will of course be asked to give the baby a surname as well as a Christian name. *You can choose either your own surname or that of his father*, no matter whether the father signed the birth register or not. If you marry the father after your baby is born, your baby will automatically become legitimated. You should then inform your local Registrar of Births, Deaths and Marriages, so that your child's birth entry can be altered and he can have a new birth certificate.

Making a will
Soon after your baby's birth you should make provision for him in the event of your death. Some form of life assurance policy may be a good idea and you should make a will providing for your baby and appointing a relative or friend (whose consent you must obtain first) as his guardian, should anything happen to you.

BE PROUD OF YOUR CHILD

Try to accept the fact that you are now a mother and take pride in being a good one. If you feel guilty or defensive that will only make you unhappy and may affect your child and may make him conscious of his status. So, face the problem in the way that makes you feel most confident and make up your mind to behave normally. If you like, you can call yourself "Mrs" and wear a wedding ring – just notify the Department of Health and Social Security and your bank etc., so they can alter your cards and their own records.

As soon as possible, tell your child about his father in a way that he will understand. Until he is old enough to appreciate what it means, you needn't mention the fact that you and his father were not married.

One of the most difficult things about illegitimacy is that many children have no knowledge of their father's identity. You may still be in touch with the baby's father and perhaps he may come to visit you from time to time. Even if your child has never met his father and never mentions him, he is bound to wonder or worry, especially when he goes to school. It will help if he is able to feel proud of his father and to tell his schoolfriends something of his history. So do tell your child as much as you can about his father and speak of him affectionately and with respect. After all, you felt enough for him to make love and even if the baby was conceived as the result of a one night affair, you must try not to let the experience put you off men in general and you must try to avoid bitterness both for your own sake and for the sake of your child.

From time to time you may welcome advice or help from outside your family. Don't be afraid to ask for it. Your social worker or a local authority social worker will be willing to give you advice (there is now a local authority Social Services Department in every area which includes social workers ready to help anyone who needs help or advice) and NCUMC is always glad to help a mother however old her child is.

In the foregoing pages I have assumed that both of you have been in accord about your choice of action and that your future relationship will at least be a friendly one. This isn't always true, of course. In some cases you may have become so disenchanted with each other that your relationship changes to hostility from the moment one of you runs away from responsibility. If this occurs, the responsible one of you can be very grateful that you were not linked to the other in marriage. An irresponsible person out of marriage is just as irresponsible within marriage. What you must learn from the sad experience is how to assess character better, how to protect yourself through birth control, and how to let love speak first before giving full voice to sex. By all means don't damn yourself or start feeling like a second-class citizen. You are still a first-class citizen, though one who is busily learning some hard facts about life.

CHAPTER 8

Sexual problems

PROBABLY you have heard a number of terms that describe sexual inadequacy in intercourse. You should know their meanings.

The first is *impotence*. Impotence applies to a man whose erection fails him at the moment he wishes to penetrate his partner's vagina. Obviously, if his penis is not firm he cannot effect entrance and then both he and his partner are likely to feel let down. All men have this experience at one time or another, but if a boy is unduly worried when it first happens to him, then the next time he tries to make love, his mind may be so distracted by the unhappy memory of the last time that the negative thought will, in itself, cause him to lose his erection again. At this point he may become too anxious about his own sexual responses, and thereafter he becomes conditioned to start each lovemaking experience with lack of confidence. Self-confidence counts more in sexual performance than anywhere else I know.

In spite of the fact that impotence is largely due to psychological reasons, many boys get the notion after a failure or two that something physiological is wrong with them, and wonder if they should see a doctor.

A rough rule of thumb for determining whether medical aid or psychological help is needed is the following: Men often have an erection on awakening. If a boy experiences this phenomenon he can be pretty certain that his impotence has no medical basis in fact and that all he needs is renewal of his own self-confidence.

His girl can help a lot by suggesting that they return to the old petting techniques which they both enjoyed together, coming to orgasm in this way for a while. Soon he will once again discover that he has nothing to fear and can perform adequately. A girl would be wise to accept the fact gracefully that every man, at one time or another, finds that he cannot have an erection on demand, even though his mind and his heart may desire it mightily.

She should remind herself that she too is not always able to come to orgasm easily or even at all, and that it helps a relationship to recognize that the sexual expression of love is sometimes affected by many subtle things that are not related to mutual love. A girl is lucky in that she can always pretend responsiveness if she wants to, if her own body reactions are not quite up to concert pitch, but a boy cannot do likewise. He must *feel* confidence and be in good shape physically to effect good sexual performance.

Any young man who suffers impotence over a long period of time should, of course, seek a therapist who understands psychosexual problems, for with professional help impotence can often be resolved.

The word impotence should never be confused with the word *sterility* or *sterile*. Many young people think that the two are the same. Sterility applies to a man or a woman who, for one reason or another, is incapable of conceiving a child. For example, a boy's sperm may be deficient in quantity or quality, or a girl's tubes may be blocked so that the sperm cannot reach the egg for fertilization. Infertility is checked carefully by a physician upon request.

Another inadequacy which boys quite frequently experience is *premature ejaculation*. This occurs when a boy ejaculates almost immediately after entrance into the vagina of the girl, sometimes even before entrance is achieved. This cuts short his own pleasure in the sexual act, and generally makes it impossible for the girl to have any enjoyment whatsoever, unless of course he has carefully brought her to a high pitch of excitement before entering, or thoughtfully caresses her to orgasm with his hand afterward.

Premature ejaculation has many causes, almost all psychological, and is related to poor conditioning. In nearly every instance it can be cured. Generally, it is a symptom of the same kind of fear which prevents girls from masturbating in childhood, and which induces boys to masturbate quickly, usually in the bathroom before their mothers can call out, "what are you doing in there so long?" For such a boy masturbation becomes surreptitious, something stolen, an act brought to conclusion in the speediest interval possible; not something prolonged and enjoyed with his parents' full understanding and approval. Later when lovemaking with a partner makes long-continued sex play desirable for his own and his girl's pleasure, his childhood conditioning acts as a deterrent.

There are various techniques for reconditioning such responses. One is for a boy to practise bringing himself up to a peak of excitation just short of ejaculation, then quietly containing his pleasure – "breathing with it", as it were – without further stimulation. When he has "cooled it" for a few moments, he may again restimulate himself, thus teaching himself to postpone the moment of ejaculation. Some boys can maintain erection for extended periods in masturbation, but their anxiety when with a girl is so great that premature ejaculation occurs anyway, to their great dismay.

In this case, a good technique is for the girl to participate in the reconditioning (retraining) process. She caresses his penis with her hands until he instructs her to stop – just short of ejaculation. This is done again and again – always ending such practice sessions with orgasm for both partners (manually stimulated, of course). When he can delay his ejaculation in her hands for several minutes, they can move on to the next step. Let her introduce cold cream on her hands (which feels very much like the lubricated internal environment of her vagina). Again carry on practice sessions until the signal for ejaculation occurs after longer and longer sex play.

When the boy can control his need to ejaculate in the lubricated hand of his girl, he is usually ready to do so intra-vaginally. Since premature ejaculation is really pleasure anxiety, coupled with fear of a woman's disapproval, the most effective aspect of such a "training process" is that a boy learns that his girl *does* approve of his maleness and of his pleasure. If she can look at and handle his penis with tenderness, reverence and love, she is counteracting the crippling influence of his Puritanical upbringing which made him hesitant and afraid in her presence in the first place. The more she can get across to him the joy she feels as she observes the miracle of his penis moving from flaccidity to erection, complimenting her presence in the most primary way a man can compliment a woman's presence, the more he will lose his fear of sex pleasure and the longer he will be able to maintain erection.

In *overexcitement*, it sometimes helps to have a quick orgasm right at the beginning – letting the girl know, of course, that this is only a preamble. Then the boy can take time for lovemaking in a slow and leisurely fashion; paying full attention to the girl's needs and responses. When she has reached a peak of excitement – perhaps some thirty minutes later, it is highly probable that he will once more find his penis erect and that he is ready to enjoy a second orgasm with her.

Another sexual inadequacy from which both men and women can suffer is *frigidity*. In the purest meaning of the word, frigidity is an inability to experience sexual feeling at all. However, the word is rarely used in its absolute sense. In fact, many nonfrigid reactions are incorrectly called frigidity. For example, a girl may be capable of great sexual response and excitement, but be unable to release her sexual tension in orgasm. This is a severe frustration to her, for far from being frigid she is quite the opposite. She experiences a great deal of feeling, indeed; so much so, that she literally explodes with exasperation when she cannot adequately release her feelings. Her full responsiveness, in other words, is blocked. This kind of problem can usually be resolved with the help of a good marriage guidance counsellor. Learning how to masturbate to orgasm can help.

Some girls feel sexually alive during part of each month and very disinterested during the other part. They seem to "come into heat" much as other mammals do. During the disinterest period, their condition seems to their lovers like frigidity and is quite frustrating to the boy who may want to enjoy sex day in and day out. He cannot understand why she likes sex at one time and refuses it at another. Usually the girl is responding in exaggerated form to the estrogen-progesterone cycle that is experienced by every female every month. Occasionally, under a physician's direction such a girl's relative frigidity can be modified by the administration of estrogen in some form. This may also alleviate the moodiness which these girls often experience. Also, a girl can modify her partner's frustration by bringing him to orgasm with her hands when she doesn't feel like doing so through intercourse.

Boys suffer frigidity also, though this isn't as generally recognized as it is in girls. It can occur when a boy has been brought up in a very sex-negative cultural atmosphere, usually by women who detest everything male about men. Often his mother has set great store by her son's intellectual or artistic achievements and has derided as crude and useless his male-animal successes in sports or rough games with other boys.

This boy may need help from a therapist to aid him in restoring his feelings of adequacy as a man – indeed, to help him feel at home with his sexuality at all. But a partner who can help him relax and who approves of his maleness is the best medicine he can have.

Another recent problem is the use of drugs to enhance the quality of sexual experience. You may have heard that smoking "pot" or taking LSD will help break through inhibitions ("blow your mind") and that suddenly the bells will ring in a wilder and more melodic tune than could possibly be achieved without it. There is little if any evidence that this is so. Inhibitions may, indeed, be broken down, but what usually emerges is the raw emotion connected with the original inhibition – usually raw fear. The resultant anxiety takes careful, skilled psychiatric handling to reduce to manageable terms. It certainly does not belong in a lovemaking experience.

When two uninhibited partners, free of emotional hang-ups, use drugs to amplify or enhance what is already a delightful experience, they usually find that their own imaginative equipment is superior to any artificial stimulant.

Of the so-called stimulants in use, marihuana is reported as yielding the most generally satisfying sensory experience (though not necessarily sexual in nature) and LSD the least, with alcohol somewhere in between. LSD used without skilled psychiatric supervision can have so many injurious effects that most young people are steering clear of it.

While marihuana may have no demonstrable long-term bad effects, the possibility of getting caught doing something illegal and often severely punished, with the danger of ruining one's future, tends to cancel out any possible pleasure from its use. If marihuana is legitimized (as many people believe it will be), it may be added to the list of mild pleasures enjoyed by man – sensual, though not necessarily sexual. It is, however, a two-edged sword. Just as in cigarette smoking there lies the hidden danger of cancer, so in marihuana there may lurk unpredictable consequences equally devastating. Since there are no established standards of purity in that which is being peddled, a user may at one time have pronounced reactions and at another have none at all.

Alcohol, which is perfectly legal, is a sexual depressant rather than a stimulant. One drink may help a girl and boy lose their inhibitions, but too many drinks can make a boy lose his erection or his power to come to orgasm.

All in all, the more you can depend on your own healthy energy, reinforced by practice in the use of your imaginative faculties, the better your sex experience will be – and the less you will crave stimulation from artificial sources which are usually not so very stimulating after all, and do not add appreciably to the pleasure.

Just as full participation in any activity is more satisfying than being a spectator on the sidelines, so is full participation of one's consciousness in sexual activities more satisfying than being separated from reality by drugs.

Venereal disease is sometimes a casualty of indiscriminate sex which may alarm you. Many moralists in newspapers, pulpits and other public media would still have you think that if you have a premarital sex experience of any kind, the penalty may be great. While enlightened people deride such scare propaganda, venereal disease is nothing to laugh off as inconsequential, for indeed its consequences can be horrendous. However, the fact is they need not be.

The word venereal stems from Venus, the Goddess of Love, and from the noun venery, meaning sexual intercourse. Venereal disease is contracted during intercourse from a partner who has it. Often the person who has the infection does not even know that he or she does have it, though usually it is at least suspected.

The two most commonly known forms are gonorrhoea and syphilis, of which the latter is much the more serious. Gonorrhoea starts as a local infection which attacks the genital organs of the female and the urinary tract of the male. The first symptoms turn up three to seven days after intercourse. In the male the symptoms consist of a burning sensation during urination, and is shortly followed by a puslike discharge from the urethra. In the female the symptoms may be painful urination followed by a vaginal discharge. Some girls have no symptoms sufficiently disturbing to bother them, but they can be infected just the same. Penicillin is the drug used to cure gonorrhoea, and it is very important that both partners be treated simultaneously so that they don't reinfect each other or infect other persons.

In recent years a new strain of gonorrhoea has developed which is resistant to penicillin. Doctors and health departments are deeply disturbed about this and several large-scale research studies have been launched to try to bring it under control.

Syphilis is a vastly more devastating infection if left untreated. In its early stages it causes a sore to appear at the part of the body where the germs enter, usually the genitals. This is called the primary stage. Shortly the secondary stage begins which is ushered in by a generalized rash, along with small infectious ulcers in the mouth.

About then, an infected person may develop syphilitic meningitis or some other form of syphili of the nervous system. Eventually the disease goes into a latent period and may be dormant for years only to reappear in a percentage of cases in such diseases as paresis (a form of insanity, commonly called softening of the brain), or in severe heart disease, or in blindness, or locomotor disability.

Syphilis can be successfully cured in 99 per cent of the cases if it is treated at the stage before the rash begins. If the rash has emerged the success rate then drops slightly, but not significantly. In the latent period the serious consequences can also be almost completely avoided by treatment. In other words, if boys and girls who suspect that they may have contracted venereal disease would go to the doctor promptly, they would have very little to fear. But go to a qualified doctor and not to an advertising quack.

Cases of syphilis in persons under twenty years of age are estimated to have increased by 200 per cent between 1960 and 1965. According to the Surgeon General of the United States, fifteen hundred young Americans contract venereal disease every day in the year. In England venereal diseases are not notifiable; in America, they are. It is recognized that the distribution of venereal diseases is increasing throughout the world. While such facts are something to make any serious young person think long and soberly, they are not quoted here to frighten those of you who are seriously in love and who have an intelligent respect for your own body and the body of your beloved. It is, however, additional evidence pointing to the fact that good sexuality depends upon your ability to be utterly trustworthy and to keep your body in a healthy state.

In all my years of practice as a marriage counsellor I have encountered only a handful of persons who have contracted a venereal disease. What this means is that where a man or woman is highly selective about the person with whom he or she makes love, and where the partners limit their lovemaking to each other, there is very little chance for the contraction of venereal disease.

What has concerned me much more than venereal disease has been the high incidence of other forms of vaginal infections which are very annoying and which do interfere with pleasurable sexuality. Little is ever mentioned about them and yet their presence can temporarily ruin a girl's chance for sexual pleasure in intercourse, and can cause her to become very irritated and irritable besides.

The two most common of these infections are monilia and trichomoniasis.

SEXUAL PROBLEMS 103

Monilia is a fungus infection and causes a whitish discharge. It often stings and burns, and the vaginal tissues may become so irritated from the discharge that intercourse is painful. It should be treated by a physician. Many doctors pay altogether too little attention to the necessarily prolonged treatment of monilia. They also pay too little attention to treating the sexual partner of a girl who is suffering from it. While boys don't suffer from these infections, they can carry them and reinfect the girl after she has been successfully treated. Then the whole process begins again.

It is difficult to determine the incidence of monilia, but a great many patients report a history of having had it at one time or another. If a girl feels itchy, burning sensations in her vagina, she should at once seek help from her gynaecologist and should not be content with temporary cessation of symptoms. She should insist on being checked at intervals for at least three months to see that the medication which she has been given has completely eradicated any evidence of monilia. Furthermore, if she is having sexual relations, she should insist that her partner too take the medication simultaneously with her and that he wear a condom during intercourse throughout the period of treatment.

Trichomoniasis is another bothersome infection. It causes a foamy, offensively smelling discharge which is produced by the trichomonas parasite. There is an anti-trichomonal drug taken orally which your doctor can prescribe, and treatment should be instituted at once as this condition is highly infectious and very irritating. The discharge causes a burning sensation and chafing of the skin in the vulvar region and also itching.

In general, if there is any vaginal discomfort or discharge a girl should check with her gynaecologist. I might say that the infections discussed above carry no sociosexual implications as do the venereal diseases, for these infections are acquired in many ways and are not necessarily associated with sexual intercourse. However, their negative effect upon the pleasure of sexual intercourse is profound.

CHAPTER 9

Sexual deviations

POSITIVE sexuality is your birthright; yet this is no guarantee that negative influences cannot cause it to go wrong. In sex many things can go wrong. If sexual expression is so far off-beat that it isolates an individual from the bulk of society or if it is harmful in its effect on others, we speak of this as sexual deviation.

Dr Alfred C. Kinsey and others have made studies covering a vast range of sexual activity. From such studies we learn that in the United States certain kinds of sexuality are normal – that is, they are indulged in by half or more of the population. Some of these normal acts are condemned by law and others are frowned on by various religions. Nevertheless, they persist, in spite of legal, social, and religious taboos, for many of them are among the sexual pleasures most valued by many men and women. Under this category would come mouth-genital lovemaking, mutual masturbation, etc. These activities are considered as *normal* in spite of taboos.

But acts which force sex upon an unwilling partner are considered sick or deviant sexual behaviour. For example, criminal rape comes under this heading. Girls should realize that in most instances they can defend themselves by swinging a fist or knee into the groin of any man who attacks them, unless of course they are taken forcibly and by surprise before having an opportunity to act, or unless they are victims of gang rape.

Rape is a crime, of course, and men who perform it are very sick persons – needing much psychiatric care plus confinement while they are being treated.

One way to avoid rape is to stay out of areas where men or

boys hang about pubs waiting for pickups. Never accept a lift from a driver you do not know and keep away from dark and isolated spots on town streets. Certainly nowadays a park is a poor place in which to stroll alone after dark. If you have to go to any of these places by yourself, carry a police whistle and learn a few basic principles of self-defence.

Every man who accosts you, however, is not a rapist, nor is every man who comes to your door to ask directions. Nevertheless, if you are alone and you don't know the man, speak to him through the door without asking him in. If he needs help, you can always telephone without permitting him to come into the house.

An attempted rape should always be reported to your parents or a doctor, and to the police.

Seduction of young children is certainly a form of sexual deviation. Often the seducers are persons whom the child has heretofore learned to trust, like a Sunday-school teacher, or a scout leader, or even a relative who is visiting the family. Sometimes the seduction is without physical harm to the child. But all too often, because it is labelled "something awful" when discovered and because the child may be frightened, not having been given any guidelines on how to behave in such a situation, he may suffer considerable mental anguish.

The seducer should be taken to a psychiatrist and the child protected from further exposure to him. The child who has been violated should know, however, that he himself is not among the damned, and he must be helped to see the aggression for just what it is, a symptom of mental sickness in the aggressor.

A very common kind of sexual deviate is the man whom we call a *Peeping Tom*. Such a man gets pleasure from watching other people undress, make love, or otherwise indulge in private acts. Generally, the Peeping Tom is harmless, but he can give you quite a fright just the same. Police take a stern view of those who invade the privacy of others.

One other very annoying kind of sexual deviant is the man who tries to press his body against yours in a crowded place, such as in a subway, or a packed lift, or any other jam-packed collection of people where he can get away with it. Sometimes this is called "goosing" a girl, but the deviant who gets pleasure from such stimulation at the girl's expense is called a *frotteur*. If possible, such a person should be reported to the nearest person in authority. The thing to do is to move away or tell him to leave you alone, and if the man continues to annoy you, report him at once to the conductor or a policeman or simply shout for help.

Another sexual deviant is the exhibitionist. He is the man (and occasionally the woman) who exposes his sexual organs in public. Many times a girl has been startled to see a man unzip his trousers in the street or in a lift and wave his penis at her.

Usually he does nothing more than that, and often in all other ways may be an ethical and considerate man. Often these exhibitionists turn out to be decent family men whose lives would be ruined if the police arrested them. Nevertheless, if it is possible to arrange it, such men need to be treated. The most likely explanation of their compulsion is that they have a psychological block about not having had their genitals (or their maleness) accepted by their mothers when they were very young. They seem driven to force some woman somewhere, somehow, to admire their male organ.

The most common sexual deviation and the one most worrisome to young people and parents nowadays is homosexuality. This word comes from the Greek *homos* meaning "the same". Homosexual in the absolute sense defines a person who is interested exclusively or predominantly in persons of the same sex. However there are all manner of gradations of homosexual interest, ranging from very slight to total fixation.

Every one of us has been exposed to the warm attraction of someone of our own sex. What we are able to do with that attraction is what determines whether we are sexual deviates or not.

Kinsey found, for example, that about one-third of all boys and one-tenth of all girls have had at least one sexual experience with a member of his or her own sex. Usually these experiences were as inconsequential as an experiment in mutual masturbation between two boys or two girls. Having satisfied their curiosity, and having developed a healthy interest in the opposite sex in the meantime, they soon went on to the more usual ways of expressing sexuality.

Psychologists today tend to feel that the homosexual may be one whose parent of the opposite sex was either domineering or nonexistent. Or a boy, may have had no male ideal in his own home that he would wish to identify with. His passive and self-negating father showed by his behaviour that women were bullies, or perhaps his absentee father, by his absence, showed that women were hardly worth putting up with.

Frequently homosexual girls (more often called Lesbians) are girls whose fathers have stepped all over their wives, and such girls, wanting no such treatment from a man, feel safer with girls, and gravitate to them.

Some boys and girls simply drift into homosexuality for lack of adequate social experience with the opposite sex, a lack largely due to inadequate parental perception of what leads to healthy adult sexuality. After all, a boy knows what another boy likes, but he doesn't necessarily know what a girl likes, (and the same is true for girls). Therefore, it is easier for him to anticipate acceptance from or even a sexual approach to someone of the same sex, unless his parents have helped him to know and understand the opposite sex. In other words, homosexuality may be the path of least resistance for a shy boy or a shy girl – a path onto which he (or she) stumbles for want of encouragement to try the lesser known and therefore more difficult approach to a person of the opposite sex.

Furthermore, his parents – and the rest of society – encourage him in his more intimate male contacts while teasing him or discouraging him about his female ones.

If, for example, he says he is bringing Tom home for the night, his parents welcome Tom with open arms, but if he says he is bringing Jane home, you can imagine what a fuss his parents would make!

So it is with the parents of girls. A girl can have all manner of intimate contacts with other females and no one raises an eyebrow. But just let the same kind of intimacy be proposed between the sexes and a shout of "immorality" is raised. Small wonder that the encouragement of homosexual intimacy on the one hand, and discouragement of heterosexual intimacy on the other, often blocks a boy or girl from attempting relationships with the opposite sex.

Furthermore, a boy or a girl may be aroused sexually by members of both sexes. It is not at all uncommon for a boy to have a homosexual relationship with another boy, and simultaneously have a heterosexual relationship with a girl.

This does not make him a homosexual, especially when the greater frequency and intensity of pleasure is experienced with his female contact.

It may seem paradoxical to say that males also need close warm friendships with other males, and females with other females, in order to develop as men or as women. Such intimacy in itself will not lead to homosexuality as long as an individual is also exposed to and encouraged in intimacy with members of the opposite sex.

In Anglo-Saxon countries particularly, probably because of public censure, many boys are afraid to put an arm around another boy in greeting or to allow themselves normal expressions of affection. One of the joys of southern European and South American males is the *abrazo*, the free spontaneous warmth of man to man with no hint or fear of being thought homosexual. Would that we could lose some of our fear of such warmth in human relations here in this country.

Homosexuality, like heterosexuality, is present in all of us. It is also present in all mammals. It is only a matter of degree that determines whether a given individual is locked into homosexuality so that he is incapable of heterosexual enjoyment, and hence will be likely to miss the greatest sexual and emotional experiences of life.

The best way for any boy or girl to become unlocked from homosexuality is to give himself or herself many opportunities to improve his relationships with the opposite sex. Take pains to seek out tender and sensitive girls (if you are a boy), and thoughtful, kind boys (if you are a girl), and deliberately make efforts to know such persons well.

In the process of self-reeducation it does not help to deny

your true feelings for persons of your own sex. If you steadfastly expand your experience with the other sex, you will find the rewards so gratifying that you will gradually find yourself oriented to the other sex. Homosexuality will seem immature, less important. Since society itself is on the side of heterosexuality, the rewards are more than personal; they are also social. You have more general acceptance, you feel a part of the human race instead of an outcast. You will feel more loved.

Most homosexually inclined persons can be treated by psychotherapy today, although this was not always so.

If you think you are homosexual to the exclusion of heterosexual interests and activities, you would do well to consult a therapist, for while homosexuality is not a disease it is a condition that is likely to isolate you from the vast majority of other people. This in itself is bad, for it tends to create other emotional problems unrelated to homosexuality per se.

I am sure that most of you have heard of the homosexual ideal of love in ancient Greece. However, on the whole, isolating with someone of the same sex and making love to him or her almost certainly involves rejection by many important elements in our society.

In a relatively small number of instances there seems to be a congenital component that does not stem from psychological causes, but from physiological ones. Sometimes hormonal therapy is helpful, and sometimes the best solution is psychotherapy aimed at helping such an individual accept his condition and learn to live with it.

There are adult groups which have been formed to help the homosexual face his problem, change it if he can, or live with it ethically if he cannot. These are listed in the appendix of this book.

Transvestism is another form of sexual deviation. Transvestite is the term for a man who wants to dress up in the clothes of a woman and show himself thus to others. Sometimes women similarly dress and pass as men. The transvestite is not necessarily a homosexual, though many people confuse one with the other.

Girls are rarely if ever censured for this, as it is considered more normal and common for a girl to want to wear a man's clothing.

Transexualism is a sexual deviation which thus far psychotherapists have not learned how to treat. A transexual is one (male or female) who feels that his body is of the wrong sex, that he should have been born with the sexual organs of the opposite sex. Psychologically he feels just as if nature had played a dirty trick on him when he was given the body with which he was born. Furthermore, he is determined to have that body altered surgically.

It is very hard on the family and friends of the man or woman who insists on having such a sex change. However, I have heard of one couple, both of whom were miserable in their "born" sex, each of whom had an operation, then remarried each other.

But these cases are comparitively few and you are not apt to meet many genuine transvestites or transexualists.

CHAPTER 10

What professional help can you get?

MOST doctors are kindly, dedicated people or they wouldn't be doctors. However, of all the so-called helping professions, they know the least about sexuality.

This may surprise you because you have been brainwashed to believe that doctors know everything having to do with the body, and so naturally you expect them to know about sexuality also.

However, the vast majority have not had a single course concerning psychosexual phenomena. They are well skilled in the normal and abnormal aspects of reproduction and in the diagnosis and treatment of all kinds of illnesses – but on the whole they are abysmally ignorant of the causes and cures of sexual maladjustment. They are, of course, victims of the very same prejudices suffered by the rest of society. Furthermore, doctors have led such busy lives that on the whole they haven't had time to swap stories with their friends, or keep up with the popular literature, or even enjoy very much of a sex life of their own. Recently the American College of Obstetricians and Gynaecologists placed at the top of its objectives that there be at least one course on human sexuality in every medical school, but this goal is far from being realized as yet.

All this may not be comforting news because what you need right now is your own personal doctor with whom you can talk over all sorts of problems involving your sexual self – and you may very well not want your parents in on the discussion either. Fortunately, there are a few doctors well trained in the solution of psychosexual problems.

Colleges try to choose medical staff members who not only understand young people, but also are trustworthy about keeping confidences. Yet students often do not trust them because they are not sure that the college doctor isn't somehow part of the Establishment and fear their problems will be communicated to school authorities or to parents. In general this is a fear you should dismiss.

Though sex-positive, knowledgeable, and non-moralistic doctors are rare, I have found that one of the quickest ways to find one in your vicinity is to consult a marriage guidance counsellor or a psychotherapist first. These professionals have done most of the spadework for you, for slowly over the years they have developed relationships with doctors who *will* be able to give you the help you need without blanching and without inflicting any rigidities of their own upon you.

You can also help yourself a lot by knowing how to ask the right questions, and by being willing to consult a physician like an adult rather than like a child. A doctor has to feel, for example, that he won't be accused of corrupting the morals of youth by giving you unsolicited advice. So if you place the moral burden on him by asking him whether you should or should not have intercourse, all he can do is say, "Don't". But if you say to him, "We are planning to have intercourse and we want the very best instruction in birth control methods that you can give us", the chances are that he will give you what you have asked for.

If he has had adequate training for this particular aspect of medical practice, he can also render other services to you that may make the difference between pleasure or misery in the early days of your sexual relationship. But you will have to be aware of what you want and ask quite directly for professional assistance along certain lines. For example, let us take the matter of clitoral adhesions which I have already mentioned briefly. Let me tell you more about these here. A girl's clitoris is her major organ for experiencing sexual pleasure. It is the equivalent of the penis in the male. However, in a large number of women clitoral adhesions exist in greater or lesser degree, and in many instances these can interfere with sexual pleasure. Adhesions occur because women are not taught as little girls to push back the foreskin and wash around the sensitive organ beneath. Girls wash their sexual organs with the flat of their hands instead of with their fingers. Imagine washing your ears in this fashion and you may have some conception of its effectiveness.

Dr LeMon Clark, a well-known American gynaecologist, has found, for example, that in a series of one hundred vulvo-vaginal examinations, ninety-two women had clitoral adhesions. In seventy-five per cent of these the adhesions were sufficient to interfere with sexual fulfilment.

While most physicians realize that these adhesions exist, very few bother to do anything about them; so few, in fact, that in a personal inquiry among gynaecologists of my acquaintance only three recognized that clitoral adhesions could be a deterrent to orgasm capacity, or that a physician had any responsibility to call this condition to the attention of his patients, let alone do anything about it. As one doctor said to me, "Unless a woman asks me to free her clitoris from adhesion to the prepuce, I don't feel I have a right to do it."

Now this is a preposterous state of affairs, of course, for most girls starting out in a sexual relationship have not the ghost of a notion about the relationship of clitoral adhesions to orgasm or that they should ask a physician for his medical service in freeing the clitoris.

You can remedy this matter yourself by clearly asking your gynaecologist to make certain that your prepuce is not adherent to the clitoris. Ask him to retract the foreskin so that the clitoris stands out free and clear.

You should understand that a hooded clitoris is less capable of stimulation. Furthermore, that if a woman *does* become aroused, the adherent prepuce pulls, and hurts, two good reasons for freeing it.

Another factor to check on with your physician is the position of your uterus. If it is tipped you may experience pain at the end of the penile thrust when intercourse is attempted in the usual man-above, woman-below position. This is because the penis hits the broad ligaments which do not "give". If your uterus is retroverted or retroflexed, you may want to try other positions for intercourse right from the start, such as woman above, man below. Or you may make a small funnel of your hand through which the penis slips before entering the vagina and by means of which you can control the depth to which the male organ penetrates. Or you may suggest that your partner put his legs outside of yours after insertion of the penis. Then he can push as hard as he wants to, but will not penetrate deeply enough to hurt you. The reason for knowing the position of your uterus, before having sexual intercourse is to help you initiate sex in a way which will prevent pain and promote maximal pleasurable responses.

There is one other thing to know about a retroverted uterus. The anterior fornix tends to be enlarged and occasionally the penis goes in above the cervix in such a way that it hits the bladder and this causes pain. In such instances, a girl can pull her mate up higher on her body so that his penis will enter at more of a downward angle so that it passes beneath the cervix. Then it will not hurt her. If he attempts intercourse from low down between her legs, the penis tends to go in horizontally, and the possibility of hitting the cervix or hitting above the cervix and striking the bladder is very much greater.

Ask the doctor to check on minor vaginal infections such as monilia and trichomonas of which I have already written (see pages 102-3). Often physicians pay little or no attention to these infections, but their presence interferes mightily with your sexual pleasure.

Some girls suffer from excessive discharge. If this is the case with you, ask your doctor to examine your cervix for the possibility of cervical erosions and ask his advice on treating this condition.

Most important of all to discuss with your doctor is the matter of birth control. Usually your total life plan of study and

WHAT PROFESSIONAL HELP CAN YOU GET? 115

work requires that you delay conception until you can provide a secure home for a child. Indeed, any relationship is usually stabilized by a period of time before conception so that two people can come to know each other in the deep and intimate way that is only possible when you live together. The more profound your love for each other and for children, the greater will be your forethought in preparing an environment which will best promote the well-being of your own future babies. You will want to choose a form of birth control which is both safe and aesthetically satisfying to you. After reading Chapter 5 on birth control, ask your physician to instruct you in the use of whatever method you think you want. After examining you he may make suggestions about a method other than the one you thought you might prefer. If he does, find out his medical reasons and abide by his recommendations.

I have mentioned the matter of thick and resistive hymens in an earlier chapter, but if you have had any trouble whatsoever in managing your premarital petting, this is a good time for your physician to examine the condition of your hymen. He may advise an incision under local anaesthesia. This will save much distress. If surgical measures of any kind are in order, the tissues will require a little time to heal.

Talk over your menstrual history with your physician. Often girls go through a profound change in mood during the week before they menstruate which can be very baffling to a boy who is inexperienced in such matters. If this change is pronounced and especially if you suffer from deep depressions at this period, your doctor may be able to help you with medication which can control your wide swings in mood.

Normally in any thorough examination, a physician will take a routine medical history. For example, he will ask if there is any evidence of insanity in your family; he will inquire about hereditary factors in transmissible diseases; about a history of epilepsy, diabetes, negative Rh factor; a family history of bleeders; a history of three-day measles; congenital anomalies; serious heart or kidney trouble or other debilitating diseases; thyroid complications; previous pelvic operations; etc. Also, of course, he will do a

Wasserman or Kahn test for syphilis, and take smears and cultures for possible gonorrhoea if you ask him – which you should. Both boy and girl should ask for these, by the way. He will also probably suggest a girl have a Papanicolaou cancer smear test, but if he doesn't, ask him to make such a test.

Boys as well as girls have medical concerns relating to sex which they would like to discuss with a doctor, e.g. birth control, the possibility of infection, the inability to control premature ejaculation, and impotence (subjects which we have already discussed in the chapter on Sexual Problems). It is most reassuring to have confirmation by a physician that you are physically healthy and normal. Also you too need to know how to use birth control effectively so that you may share full responsibility with your girl in this vital matter.

You will generally find that a doctor will want to help you both to the best of his ability. But he will be freed of his own inhibitions about giving you that help if you make it quite clear exactly what you want him to do for you. If he is not trained to provide this kind of medical service, ask him to refer you to one of his colleagues who can.

I look forward to the day when all doctors will cover all the minimal things noted. In the meantime, here is a check-list of the points just discussed which you might take to your physician when you are consulting him about your sexual self. Ask him to examine you with these items in mind and request him to institute treatment if any is indicated.

(1) To instruct you in an adequate method of birth control.

(2) To examine the clitoris and free it of adhesions. (Ask for instructions for keeping the clitoris free of adhesions in the future.)

(3) To examine the hymen. To show you how to stretch it with your fingers, if it is too thick or resistive; or, if need be, to arrange for it to be stretched or incised surgically.

(4) To examine the uterus for position.

(5) To check on the presence of vaginal infections and their control.

(6) If there is discharge, to check on presence of cervical erosion.
(7) To talk over menstrual "blues" and how they may be alleviated.

In addition to the medical profession, there are other professions that offer a helping hand.

First, of course, are the marriage guidance counsellors. These persons come from a variety of backgrounds - psychology, psychiatry, sociology, medicine, law, religion - but they all have one thing in common. Their training has included a thorough exposure to psychosexual phenomena. Most of them have served a long internship learning how to help people with sexual and marital difficulties. Furthermore, like doctors, they observe *privileged communication*. This means that anything you tell them will be held in absolute confidence.

Marriage guidance counsellors are equipped to advise you individually or as a couple on any problem having to do with love, sex, or marriage.

You can locate one in your area by writing to :

> Marriage Guidance Council,
> 58 Queen Anne Street,
> London W.1.

An increasing number of clergymen have taken time out from their busy lives to secure training in social work. Many have set up counselling programmes on sex education within their own churches. Of all the organized groups in the country, probably more is being done in these churches than anywhere else to bring counselling facilities to young people. You will want to make sure of two things, however, before you seek help with a sexual problem from your clergyman:

(1) Will he observe privileged communication? He has both the legal right and a technical obligation to keep your confidence

if you ask him to but he may not unless you specifically request it.

(2) Has he had special training in the fields of both sex and psychotherapy?

In general, we tend to think of the clergy as being the keepers of morality. As such, we expect them to be judgmental or to tell us what to do in rather authoritarian terms. However, my own experience with hundreds of clergymen is that, on the whole, they are far from being either rigid or moralistic, and they can be enormously helpful. Often as minister, rabbi, or priest, they may be the very best liaison person between you and your parents in situations where you are having a difficult time communicating. Clergymen also have a full knowledge of the resources of the community and can then guide you reliably to other professional people if you need them.

On college campuses the chaplains of the various religions are often chosen because of their special gift in counselling students.

I would not want to close this discussion of available resources without mentioning the guidance counsellors usually found in every college or university of any size. Many students tend to think of these as the "head-shrinkers", to be consulted only in a dire emergency – and that all are definitely connected with the Establishment. However, these well-trained counsellors are there for *you*, not the Establishment, and their backgrounds of education should have equipped them to help you with sexual problems. However, if it has not, at least they can guide you to other responsible professionals who will be able to help you. Like the ministers, these counsellors may have *had* to be such jacks-of-all-trades that they couldn't specialize in sex, but they will know of someone nearby to whom guidance in sex *is* a specialty.

Last, but not least, I would urge you to remember what a tremendous amount of help you can get from books. I hope you will read widely, for from well-chosen reading material many of your most intimate and troublesome questions may be answered,

Certainly, as you must have concluded by now, a great many

professionally trained persons are making sex their business. One day, I suspect, there will be a directory of sexologists throughout the land, just as there is now a directory of psychologists, and a directory of ministers. Until then, take the leads I have given you – and good luck in your search.

CHAPTER 11

What of love?

THUS far we have talked about sex and sexuality. However, sex is not one act but many, and often those that are seemingly nonsexual in nature generate the momentum that culminates in lovemaking. So if you want to create and maintain an atmosphere in which such sexuality can flourish, you will need to pay attention to many nonsexual elements.

First, you must appreciate that there are some emotional differences between boys and girls that do affect the way you respond to each other. Boys, for example, are more sex oriented than girls in the years between seventeen and twenty-one. As David Mace so aptly put it "boys give love to get sex, while girls give sex to get love." While this is not always the case, there is a ring of truth about it that cannot be overlooked.

Over and over girls say things like, "I, for one, don't feel sexy unless I feel loved. And no one feels truly loved when a boy's attitude is 'Turn it on when I want it.' " What the girls are saying is that they do not want to feel like sex machines. In other words, girls crave expressions of tenderness and regard for their total personalities. They want evidences of appreciation which say, in essence, "I reverence your existence. How in the world were we lucky enough to find each other?"

One girl, complaining about her boyfriend, said, "He simply has no conception of the relationship of lovemaking to sexual readiness. We can be out on a date and while we're eating dinner, he'll say, 'How about sex tonight?' His question, so boldly put and out of context, turns me off. There is nothing in his manner that sets the stage for love – nothing loving, in fact, about the whole proposal, so of course I just congeal and suggest that we go to the cinema instead. I'm sure he thinks I'm frigid."

Of course, fear of rejection is what makes a boy ask for sexual lovemaking in so inept a way. He has to make sure of acceptance before he can let himself go. Actually, verbalization of desire is not in and of itself bad, but it is effective only after the rest of the atmosphere is loving in essence.

A girl also seems to need her expression of sexuality affirmed as precious to the boy she loves. Undoubtedly girls have been more severely crippled by their sexual conditioning than have boys, and one result is that many still half believe that sex is "dirty", even when their minds tell them that it is not. In any event, they want repetitive reassurance that no aspect of their sexuality is ever dirty to the beloved.

Often, a deprecatory remark about a girl's body, as, "too fat", "too thin", "too-big legs", "too-small breasts", or whatever, by an ill-advised lover in a moment of jest, will turn her off until she is further reassured that he loves her the way she is.

I might add, at this point, that a boy is even more reactive in this respect than a girl. A derogatory comment about his body from the girl he loves is quite likely to send him into a period of sexual impotence, at least with *her*.

No one likes to feel looked down upon or laughed at, though sometimes lovers can enjoy laughing *with* each other over their mutual imperfections.

Most of us suffer some negative feelings about ourselves which are reflected in our relationships with others, particularly with others of the opposite sex. Therefore, and quite irrationally, we think we have to be perfect or else we are no good at all. The sentence we repeat so destructively to ourselves is "When I fail, I am not worth loving." So, since imperfection is a condition of life on earth, we tend to feel unloved a great deal of the time.

Yet at the centre of each of us is a core of goodness. It represents our healthy striving for life, love, and the pursuit of happiness. When someone comes along and discovers this core, he releases a flood of warm feeling and we tend to be drawn toward him. This is particularly true of the shy boy or shy girl who especially needs affirmation from the opposite sex to bring out his, or her, best qualities.

Thus, if a perceptive boy says to a girl who has always considered herself unattractive, "Do you know how beautiful you are?" he has literally moved into the role of healer and he reaps the love that all of us feel toward healers.

Such positive boosts to our self-esteem are quickened by appreciation in all its forms. In fact, at every level of human relationship, the ability to perceive the best in another draws out from that other something good. Furthermore, we gravitate to those who show us that they like us. Indeed, the magic key to response from any person is to find something about him that you truly admire and then tell it to him.

One of my own teenage daughters once asked me how she could get a certain boy to notice her. I suggested that she think carefully about the qualities in him that she really liked; then find some way to communicate her approval of these to him. In a few months she came back to me saying, "That works almost too well. How do you turn it off?"

People hunger for appreciation. There is no act we do, great or humble, that is not enlivened and enriched by a word, a glance, a gesture of positive acknowledgment. Appreciation pays one added dividend. Wherever it is given, it evokes appreciative responses in return, and thus is set in motion an ascending spiral of good relationship that blossoms into full and responsive sexual love. Gifts of appreciation, however, demand confidence in the receiver to receive. A deprecated gift discourages further giving.

Fundamental to both men and women is the need for attention. It begins with an acute awareness of the other person from the moment he comes into your presence. You show that you care enough to give him undivided attention. Too often, even good friends are guilty of listening or responding with only a small part of their being – almost as if they were plugged in and programmed for a known response. The element that is so electrifying between the sexes is the kind of full focus which says, "This moment is unique; no other moment of time was ever exactly like this one."

As one articulate young man said, "I want a girl who is alive, exuberant, and has her eyes open to the world around her. But most of all I want her to see me, sense me, react to her perceptions about me. I want something 'going' between us. If I am angry, for example, I want her to notice it and give me a chance to explode. Or if I am waltzing on air, I'd like her to sense it and waltz with me; If I want to make love, I'd like her to be aware of my sexual longing and respond to it somehow. Then I'd want to do the same for her."

Speaking of sexual responsiveness, most boys are very vocal about their desire for a girl who gives promise of becoming an eager sexual partner. They are very sensitive about girls who merely suffer advances. No boy wants his future wife just to allow him to make love to her. He wants her to enjoy the sexual experience, and sometimes to initiate as well as to respond.

Just as it is one of the highest compliments that a man can pay a woman when he indicates his sexual interest in her, so it is a compliment to him when she does likewise.

Boys of today like girls who have a streak of independence in them. Indeed, I haven't found an intelligent young man in recent years who wanted a prolonged relationship with a clinging vine, or a wide-eyed, dependent baby-doll – not even a boy whose ego was precariously balanced and otherwise might seem to need this kind of "superiority" for self-bolstering. It has fairly well permeated the consciousness of most boys that such a girl takes more than she gives and is far from a support to the ego.

A generation ago, a college man was quite content to marry a pretty, finishing-school graduate who had attained the social graces. Not so today. He wants not only an intelligent mind, but a trained, disciplined, and productive one. More and more boys are looking to their girlfriends for the intellectual comradeship that in another generation they might have sought from other men.

Today, boys speak of their delight in a girl who is inventive, imaginative, full of surprises, and uninhibited, particularly if these qualities are combined with responsiveness and wholehearted approval of the man involved.

Perhaps this is just another way of saying that a boy is attracted and held by a girl with whom he can have fun, exchange ideas, laugh, enjoy hobbies, and go to bed – in other words, a good companion, a good sport.

I might add that sportsmanship, to a boy, means not only fair and square participation in fun, but includes not using excuses for failure to keep dates or to go ahead with plans agreed upon. A boy surely does feel defeated when his girl withdraws with a "migraine headache" or "premenstrual tension" whenever she needs to escape from something she doesn't like.

"I'd rather she faced me fair and square, and told me what she really felt. Then we could solve the problem in some way satisfactory to us both," said one baffled young man. "I don't like to shadowbox. Besides, I'm sympathetic when a person is really sick and I'd go to any length to help my girl if she were in real trouble. But if I don't know what that trouble is, I'm stymied – and frustrated."

The question of excuses or white lies brings up the matter of truth in any intimate relationship. Both sexes express longing for someone whom they can trust, someone who is capable of knowing the best and the worst, and yet still love them.

"I'd rather my boyfriend have any other fault than that of lying", said one girl.

"Truth", said another, "is the only thing that anyone can really count on in a relationship. Even when it is rough on me, I'd rather know the truth than be told a falsehood, even a petty falsehood."

This sentiment is echoed and re-echoed. Manhood and womanhood are identified with the kind of courage it takes to be honest. Truth is recognized as the essence of a relationship, without which most boys and girls sense that the relationship itself cannot survive.

Fear, of course, is what breeds dishonesty.

"If he knew what I was thinking, or what I did, he would reject me totally", said one girl. In this spirit, a boy or a girl withholds the truth or offers a lie. But a lie is always a dangerous thing. It is like something which floats in the air, having no connection with reality. Then a framework to hold it must also be invented and this scaffolding all too often collapses, leaving the inventor in a mess. It is also a great tension creator, since the liar must always see that he says nothing that will conflict with his original lie. Even petty lying is not the answer, because dishonesty can rarely be maintained on a petty basis. It imperceptibly, but surely, invades larger and larger areas of life until the whole structure of a relationship is perilously undermined.

Couples who have managed enduring love take infinite pains to encourage the confrontation of truth without fear of punitive consequences. Each is so convinced of the love of the other, that no matter what happens, each knows there is a foundation of trust between them that cannot be shattered.

I suppose that all of us have moments when we stand, like scared children, confronted by our own inadequacies. It is reassuring beyond words, at such times, to have someone believe in us, stand by us, upgrade us when we are downgrading ourselves.

The opposite is the negative critic. Both boys and girls feel that nagging and negative criticism downgrades a relationship and eventually drives people apart.

"What is the matter with you?" asked a friend of one disgruntled boy who had broken off with his girl. "Did she beat you up?" he added in jest.

"No," answered the boy. "If she had beaten me up it might at least have made me think. But she beat me down. I like a girl with spunk enough to talk back to me when I am in the wrong, but not one who always puts me on the defensive."

A girl I know put it another way, "He starts criticizing me the moment he gets in the house, and then he expects me to feel loving and sexy ten minutes later. You just don't feel very sexy when you've been told what an idiot you are."

Of course both boys and girls like to feel that their partners will pay attention to their likes and dislikes and will show a willingness to modify objectionable behaviour, *if* the change doesn't violate a strongly held conviction. But request for change must be stated positively, rather than as criticism, and then most lovers like to respond. This doesn't mean that a boy or girl should try to remake himself in the image and likeness of the other's dream man or dream woman, for this isn't possible anyway. Yet finding ways to modify behaviour to please the beloved often determines the emotional climate in which two people live – and make love. As one sensitive boy commented, "I couldn't even begin to love a girl who showed me that she didn't care a damn about what I thought or felt."

A girl likes to feel that the boy she loves knows his own worth. Not that anyone likes a braggart, but intelligent, self-interest seems to say to a girl, "Here is someone who can cope." Without this quality, a girl is likely to feel that she cannot count on him to be intelligently interested in her well-being. If she is contemplating merging her life with his, she also senses that she, will suffer if he undervalues or denigrates himself.

A girl wants to look up to the man she is thinking of marrying and wants him to be headed toward work that he will really enjoy, work that has some worth in the world, rather than toward any old hack job.

But girls, like boys, want fun in their lives as well as work. So they gravitate to boys with a sense of humour. As one girl commented, "Life can get just too darned serious at times. The only way you can handle it all is not to be too ponderous. One thing I love in Joe is his capacity to make me laugh. Then, no matter what happens, I know that we will shed our troubles."

Girls place relatively little value on the appearance of their boyfriends. If a boy is reasonably presentable and well-groomed, and if he isn't too much shorter than she is, or if he doesn't remind her of someone with whom she may have had an unpleasant past experience, she is satisfied. It is not necessary that he be "tall, dark, and handsome," nor that he look like a Viking god. It is far more important to her that he be responsive to *her* beauty than that *he* be a matinee idol.

Boys, on the other hand, are far more stimulated by female pulchritude, and more dependent upon it.

Some girls appear to be not only unknowing, but uncaring about what is visually seductive to a boy. Most certainly, these are more likely to be wives than girlfriends, but plenty of girls are wandering about in lonely fashion speculating as to why they are never asked out by boys. They are likely to be the ones who don't

WHAT OF LOVE?

care a fig about how they look. Through their appearance, these girls say to boys, "We don't care about you", and of course the boys return the compliment.

Boys are enormously impressed by looks, and are drawn to girls who nurture their natural beauty. By this, I do not mean that girls should use excessive makeup or should diet to look like beanpoles. I have, in fact, rarely found a boy who liked either excessive thinness (or excessive fatness) or who didn't object to the kind and quantity of makeup that prevented him from kissing his girl without getting plastered. As one said, "When I take my girl out I want her to be accessible and not so barricaded behind her war paint that I can't embrace her."

If boys are impressed by physical beauty, girls are impressed by the gift of words. A boy with imagination, who is articulate in expressing his thoughts and feelings about his girl, is highly stimulating to her.

Most boys and girls, whether they admit it or not, look at each other not only as potential lovers, but as future mothers and fathers of their children. A girl wonders what kind of father her boyfriend will make and vice versa. When either sees evidences of real interest in small children or tenderness expressed toward them, it is warming and reassuring. Certainly, long before people marry, they should ascertain the real desire of the potential partner relative to the inclusion of children in a marriage. There are few relationships more tragic than those in which there is a real discrepancy of desire for children.

One hardly has to state that girls are drawn to boys who show initiative and strength, though not the coercive kind that rides roughshod. If a girl is feeling blue, she wants to feel a strong pair of arms around her and to hear the man behind those arms saying, "Have a good cry, baby, and then we'll see what we can do together to make things better."

Half the time a girl's tears are simply her way of relieving tension. A boy with the perspicacity to understand this and to allow his girl to unburden herself is a wise boy indeed. To his girl, he is a pillar of strength, and in turn she will be the first to offer him wholehearted comfort when he is in pain or sorrow.

When a girl says she wants a boy with initiative, she is really saying that she wants him to be masterful, able to take the lead. In the social world, this means being imaginative about what they shall do together. So often boys assume that all social planning belongs in the hands of the girls. Usually, however, a girl is enchanted by a boy who plans something for their mutual enjoyment. As one girl said, "If you don't happen to like what he has chosen to do, you can always suggest something different the next time. But at least there's adventure when he uses his imagination. It's his initiative that makes it possible for me to enter his world which is, after all, somewhat different from mine, and thus my own outlook is broadened."

Most girls complain bitterly about predictable boys: those who arrange every date in the same way, phone regularly at the same time, are content to sink into an easy chair and watch TV for lack of ideas of their own. These boys have no hobbies, no exciting friends, not even any real enemies.

"I'm tired of going out with a nothing," said one girl. "I could do without the fancy dining place he takes me to, but I can't get along without emotional sparkle. My boyfriend is too waterlogged to catch fire, even if I put a torch under him."

Let us suppose, however, that two of you have "found" each other, and that your personalities, as well as your sexual magnets are effectively at work drawing you to each other. How can you make sure that what you are experiencing is love and not just infatuation? No one, of course, can guarantee that your relationship (or anyone else's) will last forever, but here are some criteria that characterize love and make it richer and more lasting than mere sexual infatuation, which masks as love.

First, love is always an unselfish and outgoing emotion. When it exists, you want to *give* to your beloved. It rarely enters your head to ask what you will get from him. When you do experience his expressions of love, they come to you as gracious miracles.

Love is transforming and illuminating. It is perceived as a radiation outward and anyone coming into its orbit can feel it. This is one of the reasons we say that all the world loves a lover, which is just another way of acknowledging that love casts a warming glow upon others as well as upon you who are involved.

You feel at one with your beloved. You are so comfortable with him that your body seems to fit into the curves of his body as if it belonged there. As one young husband said to me, "Some men come home to go to bed, but I go to bed to come home."

Your senses are deeply pleased in your beloved's presence. You like the smell, the look, the sound of your partner. You are not filled with subversive thoughts of changing manners and mannerisms at some later date when you are married. You like each other just as you are. Especially, you admire each other's character.

You want to render each other personal services, like rubbing a back, fixing a meal, easing discomfort, relieving cares.

The thought of creating a child, or a work, or a life together thrills you.

You find yourself sharing your thoughts and feelings with each other without reserve.

You cherish your beloved's well-being as deeply as your own, realizing that love is liberating and that if each of you is to grow, each must be allowed to move as free spirits move. You are willing to let the other seek his own work without pressure or coercion. You really let each other *be*.

As you move about through your own day, you have a psychic awareness of your beloved that goes wherever you go. It is as if your fantasies took wing from the other's being and returned to that being for renewal. The beloved has become pivotal in your life.

In the presence of such feelings you will find that you can build and maintain an enduring love relationship.

APPENDIX A

Reproductive biology – a brief review

THUS far I haven't discussed the physiological facts of human reproduction because I have assumed that most of you reading this book will have a basic knowledge of biology. However, just in case you have not, let's briefly review these.

The penis, of course, is the primary sexual organ of the male. Normally it hangs limply down between his legs, but when it is stimulated by any one of a number of causes, it becomes engorged with blood, hard, and erect. (The average length of an erect penis is about six inches though the range may be from four to eight inches.)

A boy cannot generally control his erection by an act of will, for erection happens quite independently of the will. However, an erotic thought is one stimulant which is likely to result in erection; others are erotic sights, like seeing a pretty girl; or scare stimulants, like being almost caught while doing something taboo; or touch stimulants, like accidently rubbing against something; or pressure stimulants, like the tightness of underpants or the pressure of the bladder when he needs to urinate; or by direct and purposeful copulatory stimulation in which tension mounts to such a degree of intensity that it does eventually result in orgastic release.

Behind and below the penis is the *scrotum*, a small bag that hangs between a boy's legs and contains his *testicles*. Testicles are formed before birth and descend into a baby boy's scrotum just before, or shortly after, birth. If the testicles do *not* descend, it is important that the parents of the male infant consult a doctor promptly, for this condition can prove destructive to the sperm-producing tissue of the testicle. A man's body can make sperm if he has only one descended testicle, but if he has none it is highly doubtful if he will be able to produce children, though a great deal is now being done by hormone treatments and other medical procedures to make it possible in some instances.

Sperm, which are the male seeds with which a boy may impregnate a girl, are produced in the testicles. Under sexual excitation they are released by a mechanism called *ejaculation*. The fluid in which they are released is called *seminal fluid*. It is slightly milky and velvety smooth, though sticky as it dries. It has a unique fragrance, generally perceived as pleasurable. It tastes slightly salty. There is about a teaspoon or so of such fluid with each ejaculation, and this quantity may contain as many as one million sperm (or spermatozoa). The sperm pass out of the body through the same tube in the penis as does urine. However, some very interesting things occur between the point of origin in the testicles and the point of delivery through the penis.

Behind each testicle is a storage place called the *epididymis* which looks like a collection of tiny tubules where the millions of sperm are matured. (Incidentally, if a man becomes tremendously sexually stimulated without being able to ejaculate, the epididymis may swell a little and hurt for a while. This is uncomfortable but not harmful.)

The sperm pass from the epididymis through a long tube called the *vas deferens*. The vas deferens leads to two little pouches on the back of the *prostate gland*. These pouches are called *seminal vesicles*. The prostate gland secretes a slippery, smooth, nourishing fluid that mixes with the sperm cells, at the point of orgasm.

The stored liquid is the seminal fluid and it is ready to be discharged through the penis. The act of discharge, or ejaculation, as it is more usually called, comes about when a boy is sufficiently sexually stimulated, or when the internal pressure of stored-up seminal fluid becomes too great and is discharged in sleep. This latter is called a *nocturnal emission* and is Nature's way of releasing excess seminal fluid. Sometimes it is called a wet dream because it is believed by some to have been triggered by an erotic dream.

Some young adolescent boys wonder what their mothers will say when they see this fluid on their pyjamas, but the healthy mother expects and is glad to note one more evidence of her son's maturation.

The ejaculation itself comes as a series of quick short spurts of seminal fluid. Each single drop of this fluid contains many thousands of spermatozoa. A spermatozoon looks like a tadpole – with a large head and a long wiggly tail to help it navigate in the liquid stream which surrounds it. If the sperm are deposited inside a girl's body as in intercourse, these infinitesimal spermatozoa swim about blindly with no sense of ultimate goal. Some find their way through the cervical opening, up the cervical canal to the uterus, and from there up the Fallopian tubes where one may unite with an ovum or egg from the girl's body (if an ovum is present at that time on its long descent down the tube).

Some baby boys are circumcised shortly after birth and some are not. The act of circumcision consists of surgically removing the flap of skin that normally slides down to protect the head of the penis when it is not erect.

At one point in history there was a sanitary reason for this operation. Today there is not unless the sheathlike skin is too tight to permit it to be slid back easily for cleansing purposes.

However, most boy babies are circumcised just the same on one of many theories:

(1) Religious: Circumcision is a sacred rite to the Jews. For centuries a circumcised penis identified a Jew as a Jew.

(2) Sanitation: The foreskin of an uncircumcised penis must be pushed back and cleansed daily. If soap and water are in short supply, or if men are too lazy to keep themselves clean, an uncircumcised penis can be a menace to health.

(3) Medical: Occasionally the foreskin is so tight that it cannot be stretched back for cleansing and thus causes trouble. In such instances, of course, circumcision is a logical medical answer.

Many psychiatrists today believe that unless circumcision is medically necessary it represents a painful assault on the boy baby which may have serious psychic consequences, just as any other early pain may have psychic consequences. They believe that the penis was intended for pleasure, for procreation, and for elimination. It is a pity to connect pain with it – especially when done without benefit of anaesthesia.

Girls often wonder if the seminal fluid of a boy is clean and uncontaminated by urine, considering that it flows through the same tube through which a boy urinates. Here we observe a fascinating provision of nature.

There are two sets of muscles which serve as "traffic cops" directing fluid traffic in the way that is appropriate to its purposes. When the seminal vesicles are about to be emptied, one set not only closes the traffic to urine expulsion, but opens the traffic to seminal fluid. The other set reverses the process, permitting urine to be expelled. Also the tube itself is flushed with a cleansing secretion which contains nourishment for the sperm and aids in their passage as they swim up into the woman's body during intercourse.

A major concern of many a boy is the effect of the size of his penis on the future success or failure of his ability to satisfy the girl of his choice.

He need not have such concern, for it is his sexual skill and his ability to express his feelings of love that make the difference between satisfying and unsatisfying coitus. There is absolutely no relationship between size or shape of penis and a man's sexual power.

A boy often wonders when and at what age he first will be able to ejaculate semen. This varies anywhere from ten or eleven to fifteen or sixteen. A boy knows that he is approaching puberty (the name given for this maturation period) when he sees hair beginning to appear above the penis. At first it is downy and later becomes coarser and darker. It is called *pubic hair*. Hair also begins to grow under his arms. Generally, three or four months after pubic hair is seen, a boy may see his first ejaculation with semen – though he may have had many experiences of orgasm without ejaculation all through his growing-up years.

Perhaps we should clear up the common misconception that ejaculation and orgasm are the same. They are not – though in general, after puberty, seminal fluid is ejaculated at the time of orgasm. However, boys do have orgasms from very early infancy on with no ejaculation, and later it is possible to ejaculate with no orgasm – though this is not usual.

In Dr Kinsey's study of human sexual development,* he reported that by the end of seventh grade (when they would be aged about twelve) approximately one-third of the boys studied had reached puberty; by the end of eighth grade, about two-thirds, and by the end of ninth grade, about 86 per cent. There is thus considerable variation in time, all within normal range, when boys mature. By the time they are twenty, there won't be any appreciable differences between those who reached puberty at ten and those who reached it at sixteen.

Other noticeable physical changes take place during puberty. These are the development of the *secondary sex characteristics*. In other words, they are changes that are spoken of as masculinization. A boy's voice deepens, he gets hair on his face, on his arms, sometimes on his back and chest, and his muscular development becomes distinctly masculine in quality. His shoulders become wider and stronger as contrasted, for example, with a girl's body whose hips become wider.

The male determines which sex a child of a union with a girl will be. The sperm which he releases during intercourse contain both of the two known chromosome groups which determine sex, namely the Xs and Ys. The X group produces a girl, the Y produces a boy. The ovum of a woman contains only the X chromosomes; if her egg is fertilized by a male sperm containing an X chromosome, the result will be a girl. If the male spermatozoon is of the Y group, the baby will be a boy. The X and Y chromosomes are about evenly divided, so the sex of the child depends entirely on chance; in other words, on which of the

*Alfred C. Kinsey and others, *Sexual Behavior in the Human Male* London, Saunders, 1948.

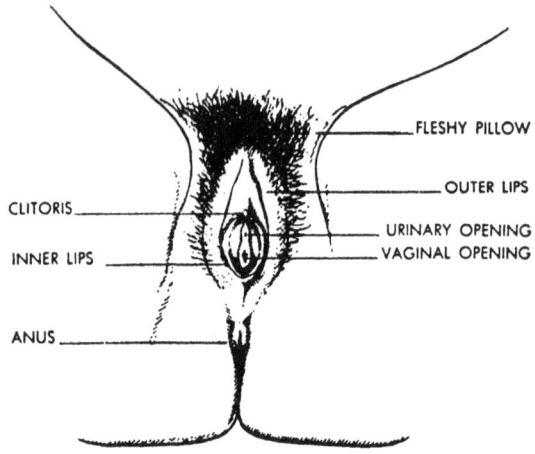

Fig. 1 Front view of outer female genital organs

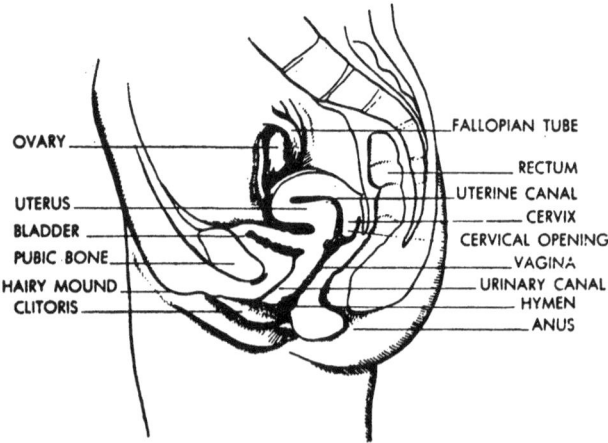

Fig. 2 Cross section of female organs

Drawings are reproduced from *A Doctor's Marital Guide for Patients'* published by Budlong Press 60625, Copyright 1964–1969.

REPRODUCTIVE BIOLOGY – A BRIEF REVIEW 137

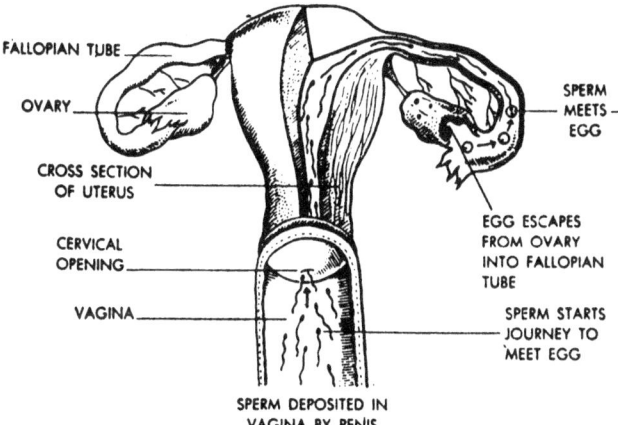

Fig. 3 The process of fertilization

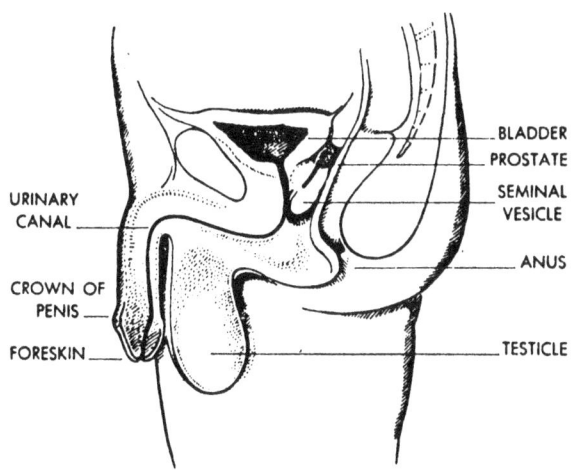

Fig. 4 Cross section of male genital organs

two groups of sperm cells happens to fertilize the female egg. Also, a sperm cell is estimated to contain about 30,000 genes. It is these genes that determine which of the father's characteristics a baby will have.

A girl's primary organ of sexual responsiveness is her *clitoris*. The clitoris is a tiny, budlike organ located about an inch above her urethral opening. It resembles the tip of a man's penis and, like his penis, is enormously sensitive to touch. Also like his penis, her clitoris can become engorged and erect under sexual excitation.

The word clitoris comes from the Greek word for key, and the clitoris is, indeed, like a magic key to sexual satisfaction for the female.

When stimulated by stroking or tickling, the girl experiences sensations of pleasure which spread throughout her entire body and culminate in the explosive surge of good feeling that we call orgasm.

Orgasm then, for the girl as for the boy, can occur without intercourse.

Her organs of reproduction are located deep within her pelvis. Her two *ovaries*, small almond-sized organs, are located in her abdomen, one on each side. It is here that the egg cells – ova – are stored. When a girl baby is born, she already contains within her ovaries (though in undeveloped form) her entire life's supply of egg cells. During her reproductive life about four hundred to five hundred of these will develop and mature.

The ovaries are dormant until sometime between twelve to fifteen years of age (though it can be as young as ten or as late as sixteen) at which time a girl begins to menstruate, a process which goes on roughly every twenty-eight days throughout her life until she reaches forty-five or fifty, or the period known as *menopause*.

When a girl is nearly old enough to menstruate some very interesting things begin to happen to her. Her pubic hair begins to grow, and to become curly. Hair also appears under her arms and her breasts begin to bud.

Approximately once each month a ripe egg (ovum) is produced

by one of her ovaries. (During the following month another egg is matured, sometimes by the same and sometimes by the other ovary, and this process goes on throughout a girl's reproductive years.)

The mature ovum is discharged from the ovary and picked up by the Fallopian tube which extends toward the ovary from the corner of the uterus, one on each side.

The *uterus* is a remarkable organ about the size and shape of a pear. It is within this organ that a baby grows and lives until time to be born. Obviously, if anything as large as a newborn baby can fit inside a home that begins as small as pear, it must be enormously flexible and expandable.

The uterus is also equipped with strong muscles that can, when the times comes, push a baby out into the world. The small end of the uterus is called the *cervix*. It extends down into the upper end of the vagina. The *cervical canal* runs through it from the vagina to the cavity of the uterus.

The *vagina* is that organ into which a man's penis slips when he penetrates the girl during sexual intercourse. It is also into the vagina that his seminal fluid is deposited, and from whence his spermatozoa start their journey up the cervical canal, into the uterus, and on into the Fallopian tubes, where, if an ovum is present, it is fertilized.

Approximately every twenty-eight days the uterus prepares for a fertilized egg by creating a nourishing lining of tiny blood vessels in which an egg can become implanted.

If the egg has been fertilized (in the Fallopian tube) it has already started to grow by the time it enters the uterus – about three days from the time it left the ovary. If it has not been fertilized it lives for about twelve hours after entering the Fallopian tube and then is discharged from the body with the menstrual flow.

The process of launching an egg on its journey down the Fallopian tube is called *ovulation*. Some girls can feel a tiny twinge of abdominal cramps at this time, and others experience a bit of spotting, but most girls are not aware at all that they have ovulated, though some feel more sexy.

This is the period of fertility during which, if a woman wants a baby, she especially tries to have intercourse with her husband.

Contrariwise, if a woman does not want a baby and if she does not use other methods of birth control, she must avoid having intercourse at this time.

One of the great problems, however, with placing absolute confidence in this knowledge as a basis for either having babies or not having them, is that the rhythm of nature is frequently thrown off balance by factors such as emotional trauma, sickness, change in climate, and other things. Married partners who are trying to conceive a child often have to try for many months before they succeed, while unmarried couples counting on the rhythm method of birth control, may find themselves caught with an unplanned pregnancy.

If the ovum she has secreted does not become fertilized, the lining in the uterus (that would have nourished it) is no longer needed – so it is discarded through the vagina and passes out of the body. This is called *menstruation* and the bloody substance is called *menstrual blood*. (The word mensus comes from the Latin word for month.) Actually there are only a few drops of blood in the menstrual discharge. Most of what looks like blood is mucus. (If you try putting a drop or two of blood in a glass of water, you will see how quickly a tiny amount of blood can discolour the whole glass so as to give the impression that the liquid is all blood.)

Some girls feel a bit droopy just before menstruation and some have cramps of greater or lesser severity. There should be no pain, but a few girls do experience pain just the same. This is called *dysmennorrhoea*. If a girl suffers from dysmennorrhoea, she should consult a gynaecologist, for there is no reason to endure great discomfort month after month.

Some simple home-made remedies for menstrual malaise are as follows: keep warm, rested, and free from tension. Don't indulge in strenuous physical activities or swim in icy water. (Swimming in water of body temperature will not hurt anyone.) There has been research indicating that masturbating to orgasm just at the beginning of the period will usually greatly relieve tension and lessen discomfort.

Sometimes pain-reducing medication can be prescribed by your physician and if pain is great, by all means secure a prescription from him.

Some girls experience a complete change of personality and mood from the time they ovulate (about mid-period) to the time they menstruate. Some doctors think that this mood change is related to the fact that during the first half of the month (until ovulation), estrogen is being poured into the system, while in the latter half of the cycle (after ovulation) progesterone is secreted.

A good gynaecologist can help a girl modify such mood swings by the administration of hormone therapy. If a girl is seriously troubled by her moodiness and edginess, she should see a gynaecologist who is sensitive to the advances being made today with hormones.

Most girls will have started menstruating by the time this book falls into their hands, so it is probably pointless to discuss anything as elementary as *menstrual sanitation*. Yet many girls and and even older women don't seem to realize how important it is to bathe frequently during menstruation, and to change the sanitary pad several times a day.

Some girls use tampons sold under various trade names. These too should be changed as often as one would change a sanitary pad.

Some girls are afraid to use tampons, but actually their use is a good idea. They are much less bothersome than a pad, and it helps a girl become knowledgeable about her own internal organs, for she gets used to handling them as she inserts and withdraws the tampon. Furthermore, it helps to stretch her hymen so that later on when she has intercourse, it will not be distressing to her to receive a penis for the first time.

If an ovum descending from the Fallopian tube becomes fertilized, it continues to move along down to the uterus (or womb), and there it lodges on one of the surfaces of the uterus and begins to send out little tentacles or rootlike structures through which the growing embryo is nourished. This is called implantation.

Later the growing baby becomes surrounded by two strong

coverings and is cushioned in liquid which is called *amniotic fluid*. These coverings and the fluid protect the baby from shocks and jolts.

It takes a growing embryo about nine months or 266 days to be ready to be born. This is called the period of gestation or pregnancy.

The whole fascinating story of the growth of a foetus (which is what a baby is called before it is born) is one of the most intriguing that a person can imagine. I would like to recommend a book which discusses in detail the miracle of life before birth, *Modern Motherhood: Pregnancy, Childbirth, and the Newborn Baby* by Margaret Liley, MD, and Beth Day, published by Heinemann, London, 1967.

The baby grows by cell division from one cell, at the time of conception to over 200 billion cells at the time of birth.

A mother can generally feel a foetus moving at around four months of intrauterine life, and from then on she is more and more aware of a growing human being inside her with a unique personality all his own.

His physical body is nourished and supplied with oxygen through her bloodstream; though her own blood never enters his body. The mother's body forms a baglike collection of blood vessels called the *placenta* which are connected with the baby's *umbilicus* by means of a long cord called the *umbilical cord*. At the placental end of the cord the rootlets have an exchange system whereby the baby's waste products are absorbed into the mother's body and new supplies of nourishment are absorbed into the baby's system via the placenta.

When the baby has matured sufficiently the muscles of the uterus begin their job of pressing the baby down through the cervical canal and out into the world where he can be seen as well as felt. We call the process of birth *labour*, for it is indeed very hard work for the mother. The labour is performed by involuntary contractions of the uterine muscles, and sometimes it can be quite painful. (See Chapter 7 "If you decide to go through a pregnancy unmarried" for a full discussion of birth.)

The baby's head usually emerges first and then the rest of his body slips through very quickly. The doctor or midwife (a specially trained nurse) are there to receive him, hold him up, clear his mouth and nose of mucus and, in a few moments, cut and tie his cord, the stub of which will dry up and drop off after a few days; the remaining scar forms what we know as the *navel*.

Sometimes the doctor will have to massage the baby's back or give him a little spank on the rump to start him breathing, but most babies just start breathing on their own.

After his first breath he will usually cry, which is the most wonderful sound in the world to the mother and father who have waited so long for him.

APPENDIX B

Bibliography

ABORTION
Abortion in Britain, Family Planning Association. Pitmans 1966.
Abortion in Britain Today, Paul Ferris. Hutchinson, 1966.
Therapeutic Abortion, Harold Rosen. Julian Press, New York, 1954.

ADOPTION
Adopting a Child Today, R. J. Isaac. Harper & Row, London, 1965.
Adoption—and After, Louise Raymond. Harper & Row, London, 1955.

ANATOMY AND PHYSIOLOGY OF SEX
Feminine Forever, Robert A. Wilson, MD. Mayflower, London, 1967.
Human Sex Anatomy, Robert L. Dickinson, MD. 2nd ed., William and Wilkins, Baltimore, 1949.
Illustrated Sex Atlas, Le Mon Clark, MD ed. Health Pubs, 1963.
Physiologic Foundations for Marriage Counseling, Joseph B. Trainer, MD. Kimpton, London, 1965.

ANTHROPOLOGY
History of Sexual Customs, Richard Lewinsohn. Longmans, London.
Natural History of Love, The, Morton M. Hunt. Alfred A. Knopf, New York, 1959.
Sex and Temperament in Three Primitive Societies, Margaret Mead. Apollo, Clifton NJ, 1963.
Sexual Life of Savages in North-Western Melanesia, The, Bronislaw Malinowski. Routledge, London, 1969.

Sexually Responsive Woman, The, Drs Phyllis and Eberhard Kronhausen. Corgi, London, 1968.

ART AND SCIENCE OF SEX

ABZ of Love, An, Inge and Sten Hegeler. Spearman, London.
Art and Practice of Love, The, Albert Ellis, PhD. Souvenir Pubs, London.
Boys and Sex, W. B. Pomeroy, MD. Penguin, Harmondsworth, 1970.
Everything You Always Wanted to Know About Sex, but Were Afraid to Ask, David Reuben. W. H. Allen, London, 1970
Love Without Fear, Dr Eustace Chesser. Arrow Books, London, 1970.
Normal Woman, The, Madeline Gray. Scribners, New York, 1967.
101 Intimate Sexual Problems Answered, Le Mon Clark, MD. Signet, New York, 1967.
Other Victorians, The, Stephen Marcus. Weidenfeld & Nicolson, 1967.
Partners in Love, Eleanor Hamilton. A. S. Barnes, Cranbury NJ, 1961.
Premarital Intercourse and Inter-personal Relationships, Lester A. Kirkendall. Julian Press, New York, 1969.
Selected Writings of Wilhelm Reich, W. Reich. Vision, London, 1961.
Sex and Girls, W. B. Pomeroy, MD. Penguin, Harmondsworth, 1971
Sex in History, G. Rattray Taylor. Panther, London, 1965.
Sexual Behavior and the Human Female, Alfred C. Kinsey et al. W. B. Saunders, London, 1953.
Sexual Behavior in the Human Male, Alfred C. Kinsey et al. W. B. Saunders, London, 1948.
Sexual Pleasure in Marriage, J. and J. Rainer. Panther, London, 1948.
Tantra: The Yoga of Sex, Omar V. Garrison. Luzac, London, 1944.

BABY CARE

Baby and Child Care, B. Spock. New English Library, rev. ed., 1969.

Your Baby, D. Rosenbluth *et al*. Corgi, 1969.
Your One Year Old, D. Daws *et al*. Corgi, 1969.
Your Wonderful Baby, W. J. Potts. Allen & Unwin, London, 1967.

BIRTH CONTROL
Birth Control in the Modern World, Elizabeth Draper. Allen & Unwin, London, 1965.
Birth Controllers, The, Peter Fryer. Secker and Warburg, London, 1965.
Contraceptive Technique, Helena Wright. 3rd ed., Churchill, London, 1967.
Control of Birth, Ernest Havemann and the staff of *Life* magazine. London, 1967.
Oral Contraception, Eleanor Mears. Churchill, London.

ETHICS OF SEX
Living with Sex: The Students' Dilemma, Richard F. Hettlinger. SCM, London, 1967.

PARENTS
Flight From the Nest, Eleanor Hamilton, PhD. Reprint from the *Modern Bride* magazine, Ziff Davis pubs, New York.
Understanding Your Parents, Ernest G. Osborne. Association Press, New York, 1962.

PHILOSOPHY OF LOVE
Living from Within, David Goodman. Hallmark, Kansas City, 1968.
Love Is Not What You Think, Jessamyn West. Harcourt, Brace & World, New York, 1959.
Meaning of Love, The, M. F. Ashley-Motagu. Julian Press, New York, 1953.

PREGNANCY AND CHILDBIRTH
Child Is Born, A, Dr Ann Dally and Ronald Sweering. P. Owen, London, 1965.
Husbands, Wives and Pregnancy, Rev. William H. Genne. Darwen, Beaconsfield, 1957.

Modern Motherhood: Pregnancy, Childbirth, and the Newborn Baby, B. Day and H. M. Liley, MD. Heinemann, London, 1968.
Mother and Baby Homes, Jill Nicholson. Allen & Unwin, London, 1968.
New Childbirth, E. Wright. Library 33, 1969.
Preparing for Childbirth, F. W. Goodrich. Allen & Unwin. London, 1967.
Psychprophylactic Preparation for Painless Childbirth, Isidore Bonstein, MD. Heinemann Med, London, 1958.

UNMARRIED MOTHERS
Illegitimate Children and Their Parents, Lena Jeger. National Council for Unmarried Mothers, London, 1951.
Out of Wedlock, Leontine R. Young. McGraw-Hill, London, 1954.
Unmarried Mothers, Clarke E. Vincent. Collier-Macmillan, London, 1955.

APPENDIX C

Some useful addresses

Birmingham Pregnancy Advisory Service
Guildhall Buildings
Navigation Street
Birmingham B2 4BT
Tel. 021-643 1461

Brook Advisory Centres
233 Tottenham Court Road
London W1
Tel. 01-580 2991
(other centres are in London
Birmingham, Coventry, Edinburgh,
Glasgow, Bristol, Merseyside
and Cambridge)

Family Planning Association
27-35 Mortimer Street
London W1A 4QW
Tel. 01-636 7866
(the FPA have 44 centres
and over 1,000 clinics throughout
the UK, including the
Margaret Pyke Centre
at the above address)

London Youth Advisory Service
31 Nottingham Place
London W1
Tel. 01-935 1219
    01-935 8870

SOME USEFUL ADDRESESS

London YWCA Accommodation
and Advisory Service
16 Great Russell Street
London WC1B 3LR
Tel. 01-580 0478

Marie Stopes Memorial Centre
108 Whitfield Street
London W1P 6BE
Tel. 01-387 4628

National Marriage Guidance Council
Little Church Street
Rugby
Warwickshire
Tel. Rugby 73241

The National Council for the
Unmarried Mother and Her Child
255 Kentish Town Road
Kentish Town
London NW5
Tel. 01-267 1361

Pregnancy Advisory Service
40 Margaret Street
London W1
Tel. 01-629 9575/6

Shelter Housing Aid Centre
189a Old Brompton Road
London SW5
Tel. 01-373 7276

Young People's Consultation Centre
The Tavistock Centre
Belsize Lane
London NW3
Tel. 01-435 7111

Youth Consultation Centre
408 Ecclesall Road
Sheffield 11
Yorkshire

Index

abortion, 57, 66–70
  after-care, 69–70
  costs of, 68
  court hearing for, 63
  how to obtain, 68, 69
  legalities 66, 67
  medical advice, 67, 68
  mental health in, 69
  risks of, 69
Abortion Act, (1967), 66
accommódation for mother and child, 89–90
acne, effect of the pill on, 44–5
adoption, 57, 59, 60–4, 84
  foster parents, 61
  order, 62
  seeing child after, 64
alcohol and sex, 100
amniotic fluids, 142
Analysis of Human Sexual Response, 28
anxiety and pregnancy, 76–9
Art and Science of Love, 28
attraction, sexual, 16–18, 27, 122–4, 126–8
autoeroticism, *see* masturbation

baby, care of 84, 86–94
  clothes for, 86–7
  home for, 88–9
back street abortion, 68
Beaton, Dr James, 45
bidet, 21
Birmingham Pregnancy Advisory Service, 69, 148
birth, *see* childbirth

birth control, 23, 31, 41–52, 115, 116, 149
  discussing with doctor, 51, 112
  effectiveness of, 42, 50–2
  emotions and, 50
  methods of: choosing, 41–2, 52
    condoms, 48
    intrauterine devices, 42, 46–7
    'morning-after' pill, 43–4
    rhythm, 42, 43–6, 140
    spermicides, 48–9
    sterilization, 49–50
    'the pill' viii, 42–6
    tubal ligation, 50
    vaginal diaphragms, 42, 43
    vaginal foams, 48–9
    vasectomy, 50
  parents and, 31, 32
  reasons for, 41–2
  Roman Catholic attitude to, 42–3, 45
breathing, of infants, 3, 7
  and intercourse, 36–7
Brecher, Edward and Ruth, 28
Brook Advisory Centre, 69, 148

cancer smear test, 116
cap, *see* vaginal diaphragm
Catholic Housing Aid Society, 90
cervical canal, 139
cervix, 114, 139
childbirth, 2, 37, 78, 79, 142–3
  confinement, 79–80
  costs and expenses, 81–2
  courses in, 78
  education 76–7, 78, 79

INDEX

childbirth *(contd)*
 father at, 74, 84
 fear of, 76–8
 intercourse during and after, 76
 medical care, 83–4
 pain, 78
 preparation for, 78, 86–8
 psychology classes for, 78
 registration of birth, 63, 92
 rooming-in, 83
children, sexual experience of, 10, 11
chromosomes, 135
circumcision, 21, 133–4
Citizens' Advice Bureau, 53
Clark, Dr Lemon, 113
clergymen, help of, 26, 117, 118
climax, *see* orgasm
clitoris, 6, 14, 21, 22, 35, 36, 112, 113, 116, 134
 adhesions of, 113
clothes for baby, 86–7
coitus, *see* intercourse
communication, honesty in, 123–5
 prenatal, 2
 verbalization of love, 38–9, 121
Complete Book of Birth Control, The, 45–6
conception, 1–2, 132–3, 142
condoms, 49, 103
contraceptives, instruction in, 70. *See also* birth control
control, 8
copulation, *see* intercourse
corona, 22
counsellors, guidance, 118
 help with sexual problems, 111–19
 marriage, 51–2, 117–19
cramp in pregnancy, 78
Curator ad litem, 63

Day, Beth, and Dr Margaret Liley, 88, 142

Department of Health and Social Security, 63
Devereux, Dr George, 50–1
deviations, sexual, *see* sexual deviations
diaphragms, vaginal, 42, 43, 50
dishonesty, 124–5
doctors, *see* physicians
drugs and sex, 99
dysmenorrhoea, 140

education during pregnancy, 82–3
egg, *see* ovum
ejaculation, 15, 23, 24, 132, 133
 first, 97, 134–5
 premature, 96–8
Ellis, Albert, 28
embryo, 142
emotions, 7–11
 and birth control, 50
 definition of, 7
 emotional plague, 25–6
 importance of, in lovemaking, 120–2
 love and infatuation, 127–9
 and premarital pregnancy, 71–4
 sexual differences, 120–1
epididymus, 132
erection, 15, 95–6, 97, 131
estrogen-progesterone cycle, 99, 141
excretion, 5
exhibitionism, 106

Fallopian tubes, 2, 50, 133, 139, 141
'Family Benefits—Your Right to Claim Them', 86, 91
Family Planning Association, 51, 68
Family Planning Clinic, 53, 54
fantasies, as cause of dishonesty, 124

INDEX

fear, as cause of sexual problems, 96–9, 120
  during pregnancy, 78
  of feelings and emotions, 5–11
  of orgasm, 4
  of penis, 22
  of sex, 25, 50
feelings, 7–11
fertility, period of, 139, 140
fetishes, 15
finances in pregnancy, 90–2
foetus, 142
forced marriages, 58
foreskin, 21, 183
For You and Your Baby, 88
foster parents, 61
frigidity, 98–100
frotteurs, 106

genes, 138
genitals, 6, 10, 11, 19, 20, 23, 42, 106, 136
  cleansing, 21
  lubrication, 23, 35
  See also masturbation
goals, sexual, 30, 120, 121
'going steady', 18
gonorrhoea, 49, 101
  test for, 116
Goodrich, Frederick, 88
'goosing', 106
Guardian ad litem, 63
guilt, feeling of, 25–7, 29, 30, 33, 121
Guttmacher, Dr Alan, 45–6
Guze, Dr Henry, 50

Hettlinger, Richard F., 28
homosexuality, 106–9
Human Sexual Response, 75–6
hymen, 24, 43–5, 115, 116, 141

illegitimacy, 92–4
impotence, 95, 121

inadequacies, sexual, *see* sexual inadequacies
infants, early care if, 83–4, 86–94
  necessities, 86–8
  orgasm in, 4
  publications on care of, 87–8
infatuation and love, 127–9
infections vaginal, *see* monilia; trichomoniasis; venereal diseases
intercourse, viii, 19, 24, 33, 51, 114, 134–5, 139, 140
  after pregnancy, 76
  during pregnancy, 74–6
  first, 34–40
  orgasm and, 4
  possible partners for, 30–2
  premarital pros and cons, 25–33
  problems, 96–103
  and venereal diseases, 100–3
  See also birth control; love; lovemaking; petting; sex
intrauterine devices (IUD) 42–3, 46–7

Johnson, Dr Virginia, 75–6

kidding, 39
Kinsey, Dr Alfred C., 104, 106, 135

labour, *see* childbirth
Lawrence, D. H., 27
Lehfeldt, Dr Hans, 50
Lesbianism, 106–7
Liley Dr Margaret, and Beth Day, 88, 142
literature on sex, 27, 28. *See also* Bibliography, 144–7
Living with Sex: The Student's Dilemma, 28
London Youth Advisory Service, 148
London YWCA Accommodation, 149

INDEX 153

love, definition of, 16, 17, 126–8
  and infatuation, 126–8
  and sex, 29, 30
  verbalization of 38–9
  See also intercourse; lovemaking; petting; sex
lovemaking, environment, 16, 22, 23, 24, 32, 35–6
  inadequacy in, 38–40, 94–103
  stimulation, 20–2, 23, 24, 34, 35
  See also intercourse; love; petting; sex

Malinowski, Bronislaw, 27
Man Who Died, The, 27
Marie Stopes Memorial Centre, 149
marriage, due to premarital pregnancy, 57–8
marriage counsellors, 17, 51–2, 98, 117
Marriage Guidance Council, 51, 117
Masters, Dr William H. 75–6
masturbation, viii, ix, 6–7, 11, 12–15, 19, 22, 23, 75, 77, 97, 104, 105, 106, 140
maternity benefits, 84–5
maternity counsellors, 51–2
menopause, 138
menstrual cramp, 78
menstruation, 138, 140, 141
  emotional effects, 98, 99, 116
  hygiene, 141
  missed period, 53
  rhythm method of birth control, 42, 54–6, 140
Modern Motherhood : Pregnancy, Childbirth and the Newborn Baby, 88, 142
monilia, 44, 102–3, 114
'morning-after' pill, 43–4
Mother and Baby Homes, 80
mother and baby homes, 80, 81, 82
  expenses, 81–2

National Childhood Trust, 41
National Council for the Unmarried Mother and Her Child (NCUMC), 56, 57, 80, 82, 85, 87, 90, 92
National Health Service, 68, 80, 83
New Childbirth, 88
Nicholson, Jill, 80
nocturnal emission (wet dream), 132
noncoital sex, viii, ix, 76
  during pregnancy, 86–8
  fetishistic behaviour, 15
  parental attitudes, 12, 132
  petting viii, 19–21, 30, 31, 32, 33
  sexual fantasies, 12–16
  See also masturbation

obstetricians, choosing, 77, 79, 83
Oracon, 45
oral contraceptives, 41–6
orgasm, viii, 3–5, 13, 14, 19, 20, 22, 26, 30, 31, 33, 35, 36, 37, 39, 40, 95, 96, 97, 98, 132, 135. *See also* ejaculation
ovaries, 138, 139
overexcitement, 98
ovulation, 139, 141
ovum, 138, 139

partners, choice of, 29
Peeping Toms, 105
penis, 2, 6, 8, 15, 22, 35, 40, 95, 97, 98, 114, 132, 134, 136
perversions, *see* sexual deviations
petting, viii, 19–21, 30, 31, 32, 34, 39, 95. *See also* intercourse; love; lovemaking; sex
physicians, assistance with menstrual problems, 115
  and sexual problems, 26–7, 51, 111–19
  choosing for childbirth, 79, 83
  delivery of child, 42

physicians *(contd)*
  discussing birth control, 51, 114, 115
  handling of adoption, 60–4
  help for abortion, 66–70
  pain control in childbirth, 77, 78, 79
physiology, female, 136, 137, 138–42
  male, 131–4, 137
pill for birth control, viii, 42–6
placenta, 142
population, world, 41
Potts, J. Willis, 88
Pregnancy Advisory Service, 68
pregnancy, premarital, 53–70, 71–94
  accidental, emotional causes for, 50
  alternatives: abortion, 57, 66–70. *See also* abortion
    adoption, 57, 59, 65, 84. *See also* adoption
    marriage, 57, 58
    unmarried mother keeping child, 57, 58–9, 70–94
  anxiety in, 76–9
  determining, 53
  dress for, 73
  emotions during, 71–4
  father, feelings of, 71–2
    responsibilities of, 65, 66, 89, 116
  fears in, 72, 76–7
  feelings during, 71–4
  financial support during, 82, 84–5
  help available, 53–7, 60, 63, 68, 69
  incidence in USA, viii
  intercourse during, 74–6
  living arrangements, 80
  medical advice, 53–4, 83, 84
  parental assistance, 54–6
  pre-natal communication, 2–3
  psychosis during, 76–8
  relaxation in, 2
  sex life during, 75
  test for, 53, 54
  virginal, 24
Preparing for Childbirth, 88
professional help, 51–2, 111–19
prostate gland, 132
puberty, 158

Rainer, Jerome and Julia, 27
rape, 104–5
registration of birth, 63, 92
religion, and birth control, 42–3, 45
  clergymen as counsellors, 118, 126, 127
religious bodies, help of, 56
reproduction, *see* childbirth; intercourse
reproductive biology, 131–43
responses, sexual, *see* sexual responses
responsiveness, sexual, 23, 27, 95–103
rhythm method, 42, 43–6, 140, 141
Roman Catholic attitude, 42, 45

Scotland, adoption procedure in, 62 *n.*
scrotum, 131
seduction of young children, 105
self-gratification, *see* masturbation
seminal fluid, 132, 133, 134, 135
seminal vesicles, 132
sex: characteristics, 134, 135. *See also* physiology
  childhood experimentation, 10, 11
  fear of, 25, 50
  foreplay, 19–21, 22–3
  and love, 1–2, 29
  literature, 27, 28, 145, 146
  purposes, 1–2, 27, 28
  religious precepts, 27
  seeking advice on, 26, 127–39

sex *(contd)*
  shame concerning, 25–30. *See also* guilt
  See also intercourse; love; lovemaking; noncoital sex; petting
Sexual: attraction, 16–18, 27, 122–4, 126–8
  deviations, 104–10
    exhibitionism, 106
    frotteurs, 106
    'goosing', 106
    homosexuality, 106–9
    Peeping Toms, 105
    rape, 104–5
    seduction of young children, 105
    transexualism, 110
    transvestism, 109
  desire in pregnancy, 25
  drugs in, 99
  experiences, first, 2, 3
    possible sources of, 30–1
  fantasies, 12–16
  goals, male and female, 30, 120–1
  inadequacies, 76
    frigidity, 98–100
    impotence, 95–7, 142
    overexcitement, 98
    premature ejaculation, 96–8
    professional help for, 111–19
    sterility, 56
    vaginal infections, 102–3
    venereal diseases, 100–2
  problems, 95–103. *See also* sexual deviations; sexual inadequacies
  responses: development, 10, 11, 35
    deviations, 104–10
    early, 3–7
    problems in intercourse, 74–6, 95–103
  responsiveness, 23, 25, 95–103, 122
  stimulation, 12–24, 35, 42, 99–100.
    See also intercourse; love; lovemaking; petting; sexual inadequacies
Sexual Behaviour in the Human Male, 135
Sexual Life of Savages in North-Western Melanesia, 27
Sexual Pleasure in Marriage, 27
sexuality: development, 1–11, 15
  expressions, vii, viii, ix, 1–13, 104–5
  and intercourse, vii, viii
  noncoital, ix
  professional counselling on, 51–2, 98, 111–19
Shelter Housing Aid Centre, 90
Social Security Office, 85
Social Service Department, 56, 57, 60
Social work agencies, 81
sperm (spermatozoa), 49–50, 132–3, 135
spermicides, 48–9
Spock, Dr Benjamin, 87, 145
sterility, 96
sterilization, 49–50
stimulation, sexual, *see* sexual stimulation
students' problems, 28–32
sucking, 3, 5, 7, 10
supplementary benefits, 85, 90, 91
Supplementary Benefits Commission, 82, 83
syphilis, 49, 101, 102
  test for, 116

tension: negative through petting, 18
  release of, 8, 9, 13, 37, 38
testicles, 50, 131
therapeutic interruption (abortion), 67. *See also* abortion
test for pregnancy, 53, 54

thumbsucking, 3, 5, 7, 10
transexualism, 110
transvestism, 109
trichomoniasis, 49, 102–3, 114
tubal ligation, 50

umbilical cord, 142
unmarried mother, status of, 92–4. *See also* pregnancy, pre-marital
urine specimen for pregnancy test, 54
uterus, 114, 116, 139, 141, 142

vagina, 22, 23, 24, 34, 35, 44, 47, 95, 103, 114, 116, 139
exercise for, 38
infections of, *see* monilia; trichomoniasis; venereal diseases

vaginal diaphragm, 48
foams, 48–9
vaginitis, 49
vas deferens, 49, 132
vasectomy, 50
venereal diseases, viii, 30, 49, 100–2
tests for, 116
virginity, 27, 34

welfare foods and medicine, 85–6
'wet dream', 132
will, making a, 92
Wright, Erna, 88

Young People's Consultation Centre, 149
Your Wonderful Baby, 88
Youth Advisory Clinic, 69, 149
Youth Consultation Centre, 149

For Product Safety Concerns and Information please contact our EU representative GPSR@taylorandfrancis.com
Taylor & Francis Verlag GmbH, Kaufingerstraße 24, 80331 München, Germany

www.ingramcontent.com/pod-product-compliance
Lightning Source LLC
Chambersburg PA
CBHW050638300426
44112CB00012B/1849